CHRONIC FATIGUE SYNDROME

CHRONIC FATIGUE SYNDROME

Living with the Unknown

B. E. Voncannon

Writers Club Press
San Jose New York Lincoln Shanghai

Chronic Fatigue Syndrome
Living with the Unknown

Writers Club Press
an imprint of iUniverse, Inc.

For information address:
iUniverse, Inc.
5220 S. 16th St., Suite 200
Lincoln, NE 68512
www.iuniverse.com

This book is not to be considered medical advice. The reader is advised to seek medical attention if an illness is suspected and before beginning any type of exercise or dietary changes. Neither the author nor the publisher assumes any liability for the use or misuse of the information contained herein.

ISBN: 0-595-24182-4

Printed in the United States of America

Dedicated to all those afflicted with Chronic Fatigue and Immune Dysfunction Syndrome, and to the Lord Jesus Christ, whom can heal us all.

And the whole multitude sought to touch him: for there went virtue out of him, and healed them all.

—Luke 6:19

CONTENTS

▼

Acknowledgements

A special thanks to my family, physicians, and friends for their understanding during my battle with this illness.

Also, a very special thanks to all research organizations and physicians that have dedicated their time to finding a cause and cure for Chronic Fatigue and Immune Dysfunction Syndrome.

INTRODUCTION

▼

I would like to welcome you to probably one of the most important texts that I have ever written. I have published several books in the past, but this one is special. As in one of my prior titles, *Living Behind the Shield*, this book also has become part of my life. The motivation behind writing this book, as well as the task of simply doing so, has been profound. Maybe I should say that the journey up to this point is what has been such a task.

Some time ago, I was diagnosed with *Chronic Fatigue Syndrome* or as it is now more often called, *Chronic Fatigue and Immune Dysfunction Syndrome (CFIDS)*. Please note that for the remainder of the text, I will normally use the initials CFIDS when referring to Chronic Fatigue Syndrome. Many of you may have or have not heard of this affliction. Hopefully, you will have a better understanding when you finish this book. Keep in mind that this book portrays my own personal experience with the disease and does not represent what you or someone you know is experiencing. Many people may be more severe than I am, and some may be better.

One of the purposes in writing this book was to help others understand what it is like to have such an illness. I realize that there are probably dozens of books and maybe thousands of papers on the subject, but this one is mine. As in many aspects of being human, everyone has their own unique experience. My story may be very similar to yours or totally different. The beauty of that is that you can see how CFIDS affects different people.

Another purpose in writing this book was to help assure the readers that CFIDS is indeed a real illness. I have read many articles and heard some medical professionals say that they were not sure if this illness actually existed or not. I am not real sure what they mean. If I and thousands of other people are afflicted with it, why is there still doubt as to its legitimacy? Although it is recognized by the Center for Disease Control (CDC), the Food and Drug Administration (FDA), and the Social Security Administration, why do so many still doubt? I will have to confess that even I have at one time doubted the existence of such an illness. I will tell you that once it strikes you, there is a magical change of heart. I will try to give my own opinions to this as you read through the book.

In this text, I do not present a formal program that details what anyone should do to get rid of the syndrome. I have seen countless books that outline natural or medical regimens for overcoming CFIDS, or simply present you with a bunch of confusing statistics and medical jargon related to the same. While there is a place for all of these in our world, I chose not to follow such a pattern. Maybe it is because I have always liked being different! The main reason, other than legalities, I do not tell you to take any particular supplement or follow a particular program, is the fact that I believe that everyone's health is their own responsibility. Only you can choose a path to follow. While I do mention what I did to combat this illness, I don't recommend that you attempt it. Talk to your doctor before you begin such a journey if you so choose.

I tried to present this text in a very straight forward style. I tend to write like I speak, so excuse me if I don't follow the norm as expected from an author. I wanted this book to present my experiences so that if I were the reader, I would grasp it the first time. Often times I have read a book and put it down feeling as empty as I was before picking it up. Hopefully, you won't feel that way after reading this one. My hook for this book basically says that this is a no-nonsense look at CFIDS. I don't sugar coat anything, and I don't blow any smoke. If something came to mind that felt right, it went in this book. I didn't include a glossary in the back because I tried to explain everything as simple as I could. It is written so that if it were me that was reading it, I would learn something without having a string of letters behind my name.

This book could be looked upon as a short autobiography during the course of my illness or as a self-reported case study. I start the book out by giving you a background on who I was before becoming ill. You may be thinking, "What do you mean...*was?*" I mean it exactly as it sounds. This illness can and did turn me into practically a different person. Don't worry; we will explore the concept behind that idea later. I just wanted to get you thinking early!

From that point, I will give you a very detailed description of how I actually came down with CFIDS. It's not that it was some supernatural flash of light or anything, just my own experience. I felt that this may help you or someone researching the illness to better understand what it is like. It may help you to recognize your own beginning into this hellish nightmare. I don't know if everyone begins the same, but it was enough to leave an imprint in my mind.

After describing the genesis of my illness, I will give you an idea of what it actually did to me. This is actually the most important part of the book. From what I have seen in other people's experiences, I don't know if the actual symptoms are the most notable points or simply what changes one had to make to adjust to a new life. I believe that both are somewhat taxing on the person.

I will also tell you what I did to attempt to combat my newfound illness. Yes, I did undertake a series of herbal and modern medicines, as well as a physical training program. Actually, I changed my definition of physical training to more that of physical therapy or rehabilitation. You will understand what I mean later or you may already know from experience.

I will try to cover some other very important subjects for you. These include the frustration of not only dealing with the illness itself, but trying to explain to others what is wrong with you. How many times have you heard, "But you look fine to me?" I will practically expand that one thought into a whole chapter. You don't want to miss that one! We will look at the impact of lifestyle change and how it affected me. To better grasp my points on that subject, be sure to pay close attention to the first chapter concerning who I was before. It will help you to see my own frustrations better.

While I said above that I would not include confusing medical jargon or statistics, I will give you the criteria for CFIDS, as set forth by governing organizations. I will also include some reference sources where you can do your own research, which I do recommend. This is not the final word on CFIDS and I don't claim to be an expert. I am not a medical doctor, and I am not a scientist. What does qualify me to write this book is simply the fact that I spend a great deal of time with my newfound enemy. As a matter of fact, we have become one and the same.

Toward the end of the book, I have included a great deal of my own thoughts and opinions concerning CFIDS. I tried to think of every question that I had when first diagnosed, and offer my own answer to those for you. You may not agree with it all, but just keep an open mind. Often times I wonder what, if anything, is etched in stone about this illness. With so many mysteries still surrounding it, maybe opinions are all that we have.

Finally, I include a short, but very special chapter directed at medical professionals. It is basically a letter from me to the doctors or other medical personnel that may be reading this book. Hopefully, both patients and doctors can work together to help gain a better understanding of CFIDS.

It is my hope that you simply gain a better understanding of CFIDS through this book. I also hope that it will spawn a desire for you to learn more about it yourself. If you are afflicted with this debilitating illness, then I pray that it will encourage you to fight and never give up. Believe me when I say that I completely understand how easier that is to say than do. Just don't let it get you down.

With all of the above in mind, I invite you to turn the page and enter a very personal story with me. Most of all, welcome to my world!

CHAPTER 1

▼

THE CALM BEFORE THE STORM

As mentioned in the introduction, I wanted to give you a bit of my background. Although this is not an autobiography, having an idea of what I was like prior to becoming ill will assist in making my points later on. While the particular events in my life may be different from someone else, the story as a whole appears to be quite familiar to those with CFIDS.

As I also stated in the introduction, look at this as basically a self-reported case study. I don't want to bore you with my history, but you'll find it helpful later on in the book. On the other hand, you may enjoy reading about some of my adventures. It's not my purpose to try to prove how much I have done in my life. The main purpose is to show you how CFIDS is no respecter of persons and can strike anyone. You will also see how much it can change a person.

Unless you are suffering from CFIDS, you may be in the dark about it at this point. I hope to change that. By the time you finish this book, I guarantee that you will at least have a better bird's eye view of what it is like to live with such a complex, but often misunderstood illness. Let's get started with my history. I'll start my background story around thirteen years ago.

I was an ambitious young man of 19 during the summer of 1989. I had spent some time in college and even played soldier a bit, but only had one thing on my mind…becoming a police officer. I was to turn twenty in the fall and wanted to get my career underway. After writing letters to the state and other authorities, I was finally granted permission to attend Basic Law Enforcement Training prior to my twentieth birthday. I believe that I was one of the youngest guys to do this! I began my basic training at the Charlotte Police Academy, which was coordinated through the community college. I graduated in December of 1989. We were about two weeks late due to hurricane Hugo crippling the state and our academy. I got my first job as an officer, with nearly ten months left until I turned twenty one. Due to my age, if I wanted to practice my firearms off duty, I had to get my mother to buy the ammunition for me!

In 1990, I took another turn in my life. If you remember, US troops began pouring into Saudi Arabia in preparation for Operation Desert Storm. This spawned some powerful feelings within my heart. I had been in the NC Army National Guard in 1986, but was discharged due to bad knees. My desire to serve the country was not gone and the beginnings of war got that desire to grow even more. Although still a police officer, off to the recruiter's office I went once again. I wanted to go back into the guard, but this time with a combat MOS or military occupational specialty. After some medical waivers were obtained, I shipped out to Fort Benning, Georgia, the home of the US Army infantry, leaving the police force behind for a while.

I found a new temporary home with Charlie company 4th battalion 36th infantry regiment on 11th airborne division road at Benning. I was to complete my education at the infantry training center as a "ground pounder" and dragon gunner. That's eleven bravo Charlie two for those of you in the army! Anyway, I made it through almost four months of pure hell and even got a letter from the pentagon congratulating me for being the honor graduate. I came home and was assigned to my unit in North Carolina, 2nd battalion 120th Infantry. Later on, I switched to the Army reserves and attended drill sergeant school. After a few years, I was honorably discharged as an E-7 or staff sergeant. Of course, my civilian life as an officer continued.

In the spring of 1995, I decided to take on another adventure. I had always had a secret desire to become a doctor. I loved the study of medicine and had even completed a degree program in natural medicines via the American Institute of Holistic Theology some years ago. I did not take the decision lightly, but chose to leave the police force again and pursue my goal of becoming a family physician. I finished my pre-med schooling and was to shoot for medical school next. With only a few years into my new dream, the love of law enforcement beckoned me to come back. It's hard to explain, so I will refer you to another book that I published in 2000 called, *Living Behind the Shield*. Anyway, I returned to the family of law enforcement as a deputy sheriff.

For the next five years, I enjoyed my return to the love of my life. I also became a member of the SWAT team and made that my new hobby. I loved every minute of it. I worked with fine people and was closest with my teammates. During this time period, I decided to write a book. It started out as a family history project and led me to publishing a total of five books, this being the sixth. My new found passion for writing was another hobby that I loved and continued to do it as much as I could. If properly motivated, I could turn out a book in about two weeks.

From books, I moved to screenplays. I had never written a movie script before, so I set out to learn how to do it. I took a few courses on screenwriting and started my very first feature length screenplay. It was actually based on one of my own books that I had already published. I had it completely finished in about two months. After feeling good about the script, I set out to find an agent. I was serious about writing and wanted to see how far I could get. Within another month, I had signed a contract with an agent.

During the next year, my screenplays were read by some well known producers and production companies. Although I have yet to make the big sale, I am still trying to this day. At this point, I had completed three feature length screenplays and six short screenplays. You can look at my current works at **www.voncannon-screen-plays.com** if you want to see what I've written. Otherwise, you can understand that writing seemed to come natural and was not difficult for me.

Above and beyond all the events listed above, I was also a very active person. I trained on the average of five to six days a week. I would run five miles on occasions, but a two or three mile run was more common. I had practiced martial arts since I was in the sixth grade, so I still did some workouts in between days that I ran. I also was into weightlifting. I had trained for a contest years ago, but since given up the Hercules syndrome! To make up for that and to keep my upper body strong for the SWAT team, I built my own obstacle course from telephone poles at home. Rain or shine, cold or hot, I would workout.

Have you ever watched the news and seen the anchor tell you what category of air the day was? During the summer months, one of our stations would tell us if it was a code red or orange day for people with respiratory problems. They would advise us not spend much time outside if it was in the code red. Normally, I would go outside and run on those days. Often times it was in the upper nineties, but it didn't matter to me.

Here we are once again. Obviously, this does not include everything that has happened in the course of my life. This was just a summary to demonstrate my motivation and ambition. I guess you could call me a type-A overachiever. Sometimes when I look back at everything that I did in such a short time span, I wonder exactly what I was trying to prove. Mainly, I was trying to please myself, but often times it seemed that I wanted to prove to everyone else that I could do all of these things. In any rate, I enjoyed all that I have done and would not take any of it back. If the good Lord was gracious enough to allow me to do these things, then there must have been a reason.

Now that you have gotten an overview of my history and who I was, it is time to change the tone a bit. What you are about to read is the change that started it all. In the past, I made changes because I wanted to. I took on different challenges to better myself. What happened next was not in my control, nor did I want to go through it. This is how it happened. This is the story of me and my unwelcome guest called Chronic Fatigue and Immune Dysfunction Syndrome.

CHAPTER 2

▼

THE MYSTERIOUS FLU

This chapter will give you a detailed description of exactly how I came down with CFIDS. It may bore you or it may enlighten you. My purpose in being this detailed was to help the reader understand the illness more, plus help anyone suffering from this illness to compare their experiences with mine. You may find that it parallels your personal experience with what I call the genesis of the illness.

It was in January, and I was to work second shift that week. This was on a Monday and my shift was to start at 1500 hours and go till 2300 hours. I had gotten up that morning feeling a bit tired. I decided to work out and try to sweat the tiredness away. That usually works for me, as I am a fitness nut. I work out several days a week and seldom every eat junk food. Anyway, I was going through a martial arts work out. I had studied martial arts with many different teachers in the past. After the workout, I noticed that something just wasn't right. I normally had a very energetic feeling, or even a pleasant tiredness. This time, I felt almost feverish and exhausted. I blew it off as poor motivation and got ready for work.

After I started my shift on patrol, I kept noticing that I just didn't feel like myself. I was sleepy and my throat was getting sore. That explains it! I was just getting a simple sore throat. I have had so many of these things in the last eleven years; I didn't worry about it much. As a matter of fact, to be such a healthy person, I was always getting sick at the drop of a hat. I started getting that way in 1991, but I never let it get me down. I kept working, trying to ignore the fact that I might be getting sick again. Around 2200 hours, it all crashed down on me.

I was beginning to shake all over with a fever. My throat was hurting so bad, that I chewed up several aspirins and gargled with them. That usually helped in the past. I looked in the rear view mirror with my flashlight at my throat. There were several large ulcers coming up in the back of my throat. These things have been popping up on me ever since I came home from Fort Benning, and I was getting used to them. It was probably just allergies or maybe some hidden stress? Anyway, I could hardly wait for the shift to end as I was miserable. When I got home, my fever checked at 102 degrees, and my throat was killing me. Little did I know that this was the beginning of something that would change my entire life.

I ended up being out of work for the next four days with the fever and body aches. Even though I have had sore throats before, something just seemed different with this one. I finally went back to work the next week, this time being day shift. I was feeling somewhat better, but my energy levels just would not come back. Being the type of person that I am, I just pushed through it. I would come home from work and continue to workout, hoping that I could sweat out this "flu". Sadly, my body kept trying to tell me something, but I ignored it.

Almost two weeks went by, and it was time for my regular SWAT training day. We normally trained every other week and this was our day. I always looked forward to SWAT days, as it was just my cup of tea. We normally would do PT or physical training first, and then do whatever was on the training schedule for the day. A typical run was two miles. In the past, I had never had any trouble running. I have been afflicted with mysterious arthritic pains for the last ten years or so, but I always kept running. I had all types of tests run, but nothing ever showed up. Using my own special way of thinking, I simply tried to push through it. Anyway, the two mile run on this training day was extremely hard for some reason. What was going on with me? I still didn't feel all that great, but now my run time is increasing? Just hold on, as it doesn't stop here.

The next day, I was to start work again on my regular shift. This was the first day of my night shift for the month. If you haven't figured it out by now, I worked a rotating schedule. I was to report on the streets at 2245 hours. My fiancé came over and stayed with me until it was time to go to work. I guess it was about 2100 hours when I told her that I was starting to feel feverish again. I was getting mad because I just couldn't seem to get over that flu that I had come down with almost three weeks ago. The sore throat was gone, but the weakness just never went away. Anyway, I got into my patrol car and left for work around 2215 hours.

By 0100 hours, I was running the heater wide open and shivering. I knew that my fever had returned. I began coughing like I was coming down with bronchitis. My arms and legs felt heavy. My head felt as if it were going to explode. What was going on? I arrested a drunk driver at 0400, which took every bit of strength that I had left. When I got home at 0730, I was spent. I went to the recliner and didn't move until late that evening. My fiancé came and drove me to one of those after hours quick care places, because I was completely unable to drive myself.

The doctor checked me out and did a strep test on my throat. The test was negative, but my fever was still hanging at about 103 degrees. They told me I probably had a virus or flu. A couple more antibiotics and I was off to deal with the problem again. The trip to the doctor had exhausted me so much, I became nauseous and unable to lift my head from the recliner. I was now out of work again for the next five days. Something was going to have to give. I couldn't keep doing this.

The next week, I returned to work. I was feeling somewhat better, but not well, if that makes any sense. Some of my coworkers had come down with bronchitis, so I thought it was the same thing. They started to get well, but I remained sick. Another week went by and I was still ill. By this time, I was getting very tired of being sick. It appeared that whatever I had was not responding to medications. No matter what I tried to do, I was staying sick.

One more week passed and I actually began to feel a little better. I was tired, but not really too bad. I started back working out and all seemed to be okay. One night, I was working out and had to stop after about ten minutes. My workouts would normally run anywhere from thirty to forty five minutes. I had to stop due to becoming extremely exhausted and a weird pain in my chest. It ran down my left arm and into my neck. It was so painful that I had to stop. The exhaustion was unreal. The next night, the same thing happened to me. I was starting to flush frequently and always looked like I was red in the face. By this time, I was getting worried. What now? I checked my blood pressure and it was elevated. That must be it! I decided to stop by the doctor's office while I was at work the next day and let them check it.

I went to work the next morning and began having the same pains in my chest. I drove my patrol car to the doctor's office and was surprised at what happened. My blood pressure was dangerously high, so they admitted me that moment to the cardiac unit. I'd be a liar if I told you that this did not scare me! In all honesty, I thought that I was having a heart attack at the age of thirty two. I won't say that it couldn't happen, but I just didn't feel that it should be happening to me.

To make the long story short, all of my tests were normal, except for my blood pressure. I now had a new pill to add to my cabinet everyday. Even this angered me because I had spent so many years working out and eating right. What good has it done? The moral of the story is that some afflictions can be inherited and there is little that you can do about it. They also decided to test me for *mononucleosis* while in the hospital. It seems that the doctors were more concerned with me being sick for so long. For those of you that don't know, mononucleosis or mono, is an infectious disease that tends to strike teenagers more often than adults. It can be spread by contact, thus it has been called the "kissing disease" in the past. Although, not an official medical definition, mono is basically like have a bad flu for six or more weeks. It can affect your spleen and liver, so rest is extremely important if you come down with this.

Since my symptoms mimicked mono, it was probably a wise test to order for me. I had to wait about five days to get the results, so I took it easy until then. I was still out of work at this point. I still didn't feel any better. I went back to the doctor at the end of the week and was given my results.

Sure enough, I had tested positive for something called the Epstein-Barr Virus or EBV. My test showed that I either had a chronic active infection or a reactivated infection. From what I understand, EBV is the culprit behind mono. We will discuss this one more later. Anyway, I was told that I had mono. In a way, I was relieved that someone had given me an answer. It made perfect sense. I fit the criteria for it and had tested positive for the Epstein-Barr. Now, I just had to rest for another six weeks and I would be well. At least that is what I thought.

At that point, my symptoms included extreme fatigue, headaches, recurrent sore throats, stomach problems, dizziness, shortness of breath, chest pains, aching muscles, and just a general sense of ill being. I tried to rest as much as I could, but the will to get better just kept getting in the way. About three weeks later, I decided to do some work around the house. I didn't do much, just helped a guy put a new door in our Florida room. I guess I was on my feet for about four solid hours. It was hot outside, and the heat really got to me. That night, my fever shot back up to 103 degrees and it all started again. It was like I was getting completely ill all over again.

The next morning, I was off to the doctor again. I told him what had happened and he advised me that I was just still sick with the mono. He put me out of work for another two weeks. He warned me about CFIDS. I really didn't know that much about it, but I was told that mono could turn into it. I didn't worry too much about that. I was supposed to have gone back to work three days from now, but that went out with the wash. It was back to my favorite recliner again. You have to understand that I did not want to rest. I had put too much on hold. There was too much to do, plus I was missing work. Unfortunately, my body wouldn't let me do anything. Besides, the mono will go away soon. It was just lingering a little longer than normal.

Two weeks went by and I returned to see my primary care physician. I was still sick. I have now been sick for three solid months, with no improvement. As a matter of fact, I was getting worse. It was getting hard to even get out of the bed in the mornings. My arms and legs were starting to weigh a ton. I couldn't tolerate heat or bright lights anymore. My doctor was concerned as the mono should have decreased in severity by now, if not been totally gone. I was sent to an infectious disease specialist a few weeks later for a myriad of tests.

At my first visit to the infectious diseases specialist, I donated a large amount of blood. The amount of diseases I was tested for were enormous. The greatest problem was the fact that it was going to take about two weeks for me to get all of my results. This was going to be the longest wait in history for me! I knew that I was sick, but what with? It scared me to death when my doctor told me that I should have already been over the mono. So many worries began to go through my head. The worst part is the fact that I was still sick and dealing with stress while sick is no fun.

During the two weeks that I waited on the results, I was becoming worried. I had now gone from thinking I had mono, to dreaming up all sorts of diseases. Did I have cancer or Lupus? Was this how it starts when you have a terminal illness? The thought of it all was almost as bad as the illness itself. Anyway, I waited and the day finally came to go back for the results.

On that faithful morning, my fiancé and I walked down the cold hallway of the Infectious Diseases Center in my hometown. I am not sure who was more worried. On my first visit, the doctor made it clear that he needed to rule out many different illnesses in order to narrow it down. I won't list everything that I was tested for, but needless to say, many were terminal. He had told me that my symptoms mimicked several of these. That didn't help me to feel any better, but I had to know.

We sat down in the waiting area and I began to thumb through some of the brochures that lay upon the end table. Theses brochures obviously introduced new patients to their afflictions. Upon reading several of them, it didn't take a brain surgeon to know that my symptoms were indeed practically identical to many. I wasn't feeling well to begin with, now I really felt awful! We actually only waited for about ten minutes for the nurse to come get me, but it seemed like a thousand years. She finally came and took me down the hall. My fiancé was looking at me as if I were being led off to execution.

The nurse was very pleasant and warm. She took my vital signs and advised me that the doctor would be in shortly. Great, another wait! As I sat alone on the cold table, I looked around the room through my blurry eyes. I could see charts on the walls that explained different medicines used to treat terminal illnesses. I wondered which one I would be taking after leaving here today.

If you haven't figured it out by now, I was totally convinced that I had a terminal illness. The mono theory didn't work with me anymore, as it just wouldn't go away. The symptoms that I had suffered with for months now were becoming very testing upon my will. I felt like I was dying. I continued to wait and tried not to let my mind wonder anymore than it already was.

After a few minutes, the doctor entered the room carrying my medical file. He too was a very pleasant and knowledgeable gentleman. He shakes my hand and takes a seat next to the examination table, where I sat shivering. He opens the file folder, which contained all of my long awaited test results. He advised me that he wanted to go over the results with me in detail. I was still not relaxed.

He flips through my chart and test files, while wrinkling his forehead. He then shows me each test result and explains exactly what it tested for. Then the good news came, all of my tests were within normal ranges. The only test that even remotely showed positive was the test I had in the hospital that showed the Epstein-Barr Virus profiles. I was totally relieved! The good Lord was indeed watching after me once again! Then reality set in. What *is* wrong with me? My tests were normal, no cancers, Lupus, HIV, or any abnormal infections other than the EBV profiles, which he told me not to worry about. Evidently, that particular test can bring various opinions as to what is and what is not bad.

The doctor told me that the bad news was that he didn't know how to make me better. On the other hand, he handed me a booklet describing Chronic Fatigue Syndrome. He asked me if I knew much about this illness, and I told him that I knew very little. He explained that I fit the criteria set forth for the purpose of diagnosing such an illness and that he was going to make that his official diagnosis. At this point, it had taken nearly four months for me to feel like I was finally given some understanding of what was wrong with me. Don't get me wrong, my doctors were doing everything that they could and their prior diagnoses were well within being acceptable. So now I knew.

After studying up on the subject, I found that I certainly did fit the profile of someone with CFIDS. It was like reading an instruction sheet for me (batteries not included!), when I read case studies of other patients. I felt in my heart that this was definitely what I was suffering from and got some peace with that. Now there was just one more problem. What do I do about it? It is at this point that all patients come together as having something in common. Most doctors will be honest with you and explain that they don't have an answer yet. I understand that, but what am I going to do?

I hope you will continue to read, as the next chapter begins my answer to the above question. I will tell you that you cannot answer it in five words or less! This is the point where my new life began. Sure, since I had been sick, my life had already changed, but now I knew what I was facing. I was told to expect to possibly be sick for years or the rest of my life. I was also told that it could simply go away, but when? There were so many questions that I had about CFIDS, but no one to answer them all. This started my own research journey. In the next chapter, I will tell you what I found.

CHAPTER 3

▼

DEFINING CHRONIC FATIGUE SYNDROME

I probably should have started the book off with this chapter, but I wanted to give you some background first. I felt that this would help you to better understand the more formal definitions of CFIDS. So, let's get the formalities out of the way before we proceed.

So far, we have mentioned this illness numerous times, and I have described how I felt as it began its ugly course with me. As mentioned in this text, CFIDS seems to have many faces. It appears to affect people in varying degrees of severity, as well as in the actual symptoms that manifest themselves. Having that in mind, you may still have plenty of questions. Don't feel bad, as you are not alone. I still don't understand it and apparently the medical community still battles for information. The main questions that motivate this chapter are simple. What exactly is the definition of Chronic Fatigue and Immune Dysfunction Syndrome? What criteria does one need to meet in order to begin a possible diagnosis?

As I have and will mention many times in this book, I am not a medical doctor and do not claim to be offering the reader any medical advice. If you suspect that you are ill, then my advice is to seek medical attention promptly. This chapter is not the final authority on CFIDS, and I do not claim to list or know everything that there is about it. It is my hope that this book will inspire you to do your own study and learn more about it. Otherwise, we will look at what I found while researching myself.

CFIDS is recognized by the Center for Disease Control and Prevention (CDC), the Food and Drug Administration (FDA), and other organizations as a disease. They are aware that it can and often does becoming quite disabling, along with being very complex. Although no specific testing or treatment protocol has been set forth, it is still recognized. That wasn't always the case. In 1994, some experts at the CDC came up with an official definition or criteria for this disease. Keep in mind that CFIDS had been around longer than that.

Even the name isn't without controversy. Since I began studying up on this complex disorder, I have found it called several different names. The most used is CFIDS, but it is also known as myalgic encephalomyelitis or ME. As with the contradicting opinions on what causes this disorder, the name is even debated upon. I even read an article where it was referred to as AIDS minor. For our purposes, and since it is generally acceptable, we'll stick with CFIDS for now.

According to the CDC, to be diagnosed with Chronic Fatigue and Immune Dysfunction Syndrome, you basically have to meet two major criteria. I will try to explain these the best that I know how. The first is the fact that you must be suffering from severe fatigue that is not relieved by rest for six months or more. In other words, although everyone experiences fatigue, this fatigue has to be somewhat unusual. You can't sleep to make it go away, and it actually interferes with your daily activities.

The next aspect is that you must have at least four or more of the symptoms they list. These include short term memory or concentration problems, recurring sore throats, very poor sleep, tiredness after exerting yourself that lasts for a day or more, joint and muscle pains, unusual headaches that appear to come in a different pattern, and sore/swollen lymph nodes. While these aren't copied word for word, I would advise you to contact your doctor or the CDC for official information. Anyway, you should have the idea.

Now, they also tell us that these symptoms must basically be present since the onset of the fatigue and not before. In other words, if you develop all of the criteria at the same time and it persists for at least six or more months, then you could be a candidate. From that point, your doctor would have to rule out other medical problems or other underlying causes that could mimic the same type of symptoms. As my specialist told me, many different illnesses can cause the same symptoms. Therefore, it is only common sense to rule out the others first. That is why you have to seek medical attention. Do not diagnose yourself!

It is also notable to mention here that the above symptoms are by no means the only things that can manifest during the course of CFIDS. From experience, I can tell you that I have several other symptoms that began since the onset of my illness that are not listed above. It does appear that this complex illness can vary a great deal from person to person.

Does anyone know what causes it? From what I have read, the answer is still no. Unless there has been some breakthrough that I am unaware of, no one has been able to put the blame on any one virus or substance that could cause it. I was told by one doctor that it could be like a chronic Epstein-Barr infection. On the other side of that coin, I have been told that theory has since been debunked. I have read that it could be anything from a post viral syndrome to an exposure to chemicals. Being a veteran from the Desert Storm era, I have heard that it could have been caused by vaccinations and a variety of other exposures.

The fact remains that there is little written in stone about this illness. For those of us who suffer from it, that is bad news. Granted, I am not going to sit here and try to blame the medical community for what they have or have not done. Just like everyone else with this disease, I simply would love to have some answers. You may find that once you get involved with others who suffer from it, they tend to be doing their own research very often. This brings up a funny point. I have heard people say that CFIDS was a psychosomatic illness. It seems to me that most of those suffering from it are pretty level headed. They are going out and trying to study and learn more about what they suffer from. They appear to be some of the most ambitious and motivated people that I have seen!

In conclusion, there are several points that I wish to make. First of all, you can see that this is one of the shortest chapters in my book. I tend to look at that point as somewhat symbolic. Can anyone truly define CFIDS? Until there is more research done, which is needed greatly, this chapter probably will remain the shortest. Even as a patient myself, I cannot easily explain to you what it is that I suffer from. I will try to do so in this book, but I learn something new everyday.

The next point that I want to make clear is that should you be experiencing anything similar to what is listed herein, seek out the proper medical authority immediately. If you do receive a diagnosis of CFIDS, then it may be wise to seek a physician that has experience with it. From my own experience, it is most helpful to have a doctor that is sympathetic to your illness. Just remember that there are still many doctors out there that are uncomfortable in diagnosing CFIDS. Why? I don't know, except for the fact that it seems to be a difficult one to pin down.

Finally, you should know that not everyone responds to this illness in the exact same way. The description of my own symptoms in this text may be totally different than what you experience. It was simply my hope that sharing this with others may help someone not feel so alone in a private hell. Think of how difficult it is for someone to be suffering from a very real disorder, only to find that no one believes you? Stay with me as I take you into the next chapter. There you will see exactly how it changed my life.

CHAPTER 4

▼

THE NEW ME

The title of this chapter is an understatement. Little did I know that when I came down with this unusual illness that my life would change so much. For all practical purposes, it seemed that my old self was dead and a new person had emerged. Unfortunately, I didn't care for this one too much. I now had an official diagnosis and a long battle ahead. Actually, my life had already changed, but now it just seemed a bit more official. The fact that I had been told that there was no known treatment, didn't help much.

Although I had already found my physical limitations within the last few months, they really started to become a reality. That is what I plan to discuss in this chapter. Even if the beginning of your illness was different, you may find that we have some things in common during the course of this chapter. We will look at both my physical and mental limitations, as well as the frustration of having such.

If you paid much attention to the chapter on my background, you should be able to see the impact that CFIDS had upon me personally. That is why I told you that my history would be important earlier. Look at it as sort of a control group to compare my current situation to. For those of you afflicted with CFIDS, you should completely understand. For those of you who have not had the pleasure of meeting this horrid entity, I hope that you will try to grasp what it is like. Let's proceed on with my story.

As stated above, my life had already changed prior to being diagnosed. I had been sick for months before finding the cause. Let me start by saying that I was sick because I was sick, not because I was told that I was ill. Too often, I have heard people say, "don't believe everything those doctors tell you." I'm not stupid, and neither are all doctors, but these folks made it sound like that the only reason I was sick was because someone was telling me that I was. This was real, and not in my head. Sorry if I am going off on a tangent, as we will dedicate a whole chapter to that thought later. But for now, let's capitalize on the fact that I had begun a lifestyle change.

Keep in mind that the first few months of the illness, I was in and out of bed. This was the most difficult, as it was the initial onset. The high fevers, bronchitis, and sore throats pretty much incapacitated me one hundred percent. After that began to subside, the *flu-ish* feeling remained. I hadn't really worried much about a lifestyle change up until this point. You know how it is, if you get the flu, you are down for a while, but things eventually go back to normal. Here is where it all takes a turn. I wasn't getting better.

Pretty soon, I realized that it wasn't just going to go away after a few weeks. I was hopeful, but that soon became a shattered dream. After the initial onset was over, I had the desire to start rehabilitating myself. I wanted to go back to being exactly the way that I was. With my history in mind, you could understand that I am not the one to simply give up. Normally, my idea of getting well is to buy a new pair of running shoes and go pound out three miles, sweating the illness away. For the first time in my life, that wasn't going to work. Believe me when I say this, because I tried over and over again.

I believe the first change that I noticed in my life was the fact that endurance was a thing of the past. I would walk to the mailbox and return out of breath. I would get in the floor, tossing a ball to my cat, and have to sit down exhausted. If I stood in one spot too long, such as talking to a friend, I would get lightheaded and exhausted. If I lifted anything, such as a garbage bag, it felt as if it weighed a ton. I would go to the grocery store and find it hard to carry the little plastic basket around. No offense to anyone else, but to someone like me, this was degrading. I mean, a former US Army infantryman, drill sergeant, SWAT cop, who cannot carry the stupid little grocery basket around without getting exhausted! I can most certainly say that this was not in my head.

I think what really made me angry was the fact that this all happened within a short amount of time. Barely three months ago, I was a hardcore SWAT team member and a fitness nut. Oh yes, I ate right, exercised everyday, and took my supplements. I wasn't supposed to be sick, but I was. I had finally met my match, and I couldn't even see, touch, or hear it. It was my invisible waterloo.

So now, I had to learn my limitations when it came to muscular and cardiovascular endurance. I had never really had any such limitations, so it was quite inconvenient. In the past, there was nothing that I could not do physically. Sure, I was battling an arthritic condition, but I didn't even let that stop me. As I told my doctor, CFIDS is worse than arthritis in my opinion. I had to begin planning my activities around how much strength I had on that particular day.

There were good days and bad days, but the endurance aspect seemed to never change. I tried everyday to walk or jog in a circle that I had laid out behind my house. It exhausted me and made me sick every time that I tried, but I kept pushing. The sad part was that I never showed any improvement. I was used to training hard and seeing my run time drop as I got into better shape. Now, nothing would change. I could make it for a few measly minutes before I had to stop. In all of my years with the military and SWAT, I never fell out of a run. Now, it is a common occurrence. Of course, in the military we would run six or more miles at a time. I was now struggling to walk a hundred yards.

Still discussing the aspect of endurance, I can honestly say that I lost at least sixty percent of my normal abilities. That sounds like an exaggeration, but it is more fact that you may know. Now remember, along with the loss of strength and such; keep in mind that I was feeling physically sick all of the time. Being weak was just one symptom, but that is what I wanted to isolate for now. Imagine losing all of your strength, plus feeling like you have some sort of super flu twenty four hours a day. Even then, I don't believe that it describes it accurately.

To more accurately describe my loss of strength, I will give you an idea of what I was able to do prior to becoming ill. I don't want this to sound like I am bragging, but to merely demonstrate the severity of this disorder. Keep in mind that the following physical fitness scores were average for me at the age of thirty two. Should we go back in time to my days in the US Army, you could add a considerable amount to the figures below. For example, I was commonly able to do a maximum average of around fifty to sixty push ups per minute. In the realm of hip flexor strength, I could do an average of about eighty plus sit ups in two minutes. A moderately paced two mile run could be done in about sixteen minutes. On a good day, I could probably do about ten dead hang pull ups (palms facing away). For your reference, my body weight was 216 and my height is 6' 1".

Here again, the above figures are certainly not that of a marathon runner or professional athlete, but that of a thirty two year old SWAT officer. All in all, there are probably many average males that still could not do the above. Anyway, my current ability would lie within the fifty percent loss range. In other words, sixty push ups has now turned into twenty five on a good day. Eighty sit ups has been reduced to about forty. Ten dead hang pull ups has been reduced to a maximum of three, and the two mile run is practically non-existent. Of course, I am still trying to develop cardiovascular endurance by walking and slow jogging. Currently, I am lucky if I can slow jog for a total of four minutes. Also, keep in mind that after doing any of the above, and certainly not at the same time, I become totally exhausted and require up to two hours of sleep immediately following the activity.

Along with becoming phenomenally fatigued, there is also a worsening of the other symptoms mentioned herein. It is almost like clockwork how activity worsens the symptoms of CFIDS. Before you think it, let me tell you that neither I nor anyone else convinced me of that, but I found it out on my own. Prior to becoming ill, physical training gave me energy. Now, any physical activity causes fatigue that is not relieved by sleep, plus an increase in the severity of my other symptoms.

You may be thinking that the loss of the ability to do "x" amount of push ups or sit ups should not cause a change in anyone's life.

Most folks don't care to them anyway! For you it may not mean much, to me it meant the loss of my SWAT team membership, which was my life. This disease has cost me everything from my career to my own personal satisfaction of enjoying physical fitness.

While we are on the subject, let's look at the other symptoms and how they changed my life. The feeling that you have the flu twenty four hours a day should be self explanatory. Maybe this should fall under the endurance category, but I felt it deserved a paragraph of its own. Have you ever had the flu? You know the aches, headaches, fever, and general malaise? How about feeling like this constantly? That can get pretty tiresome. This alone caused me to learn how to cancel social, professional, and personal events. You just don't feel like doing anything anymore. I was quite active and never really sat still for a moment. I now found plenty of time to crash in my recliner and watch some television show that turned my stomach. I didn't want to do this, but it was all that I could do on some days.

Along with the above, there were frequent bouts with gastrointestinal disorders. Foods that once were my favorites, now hit my stomach like a bag of cement. There were days filled with the excitement of diarrhea and days with constipation. Heartburn was becoming a friend of mine, and Zantac® tablets were an after dinner mint. It seemed like my whole system was shutting down. I still felt like I was dying.

Sore throats are never fun. I used to get them pretty regularly, but never like they are now. I guess I use the term sore rather lightly. I am speaking of large ulcers in the back of the throat. I have had over six occurrences of these within the last six months. Imagine how a fever blister feels on the lip or tongue. Now, try to imagine a half dozen of them on the roof of your mouth and back of the throat. I don't have to tell you what it feels like to eat. These are a common problem with me now and I must say that they rank high on my list of most painful symptoms.

This illness is certainly not without effect on cognitive function. Don't worry, I am not going to give you an MRI read out and try to fill you up with long words or statistics! I am simply talking about what it has done to me and probably many others. Most CFIDS patients call it "brain fog". I guess that this is probably the most aggravating and certainly can be the most frightening symptom of them all. I have read some articles that suggested that this too had nothing to do with the so called CFIDS and that the person must have some underlying psychological disorder.

Having been a law enforcement officer for many years, plus an author of several books and screenplays, I was used to having a very clear head. Decision making was my job, and sometimes they were life and death decisions. I was also blessed with having creative thoughts flow through my head and onto paper to create books and scripts. Writers block was not very common with me. On the average, I could write a book in about two weeks or less. I wrote my first feature length screenplay and signed with an agent within three months. Not the qualities of one with a psychological problem.

From my own experience, brain fog could be compared to a television set that sometimes loses clear reception. In other words, you know that you are not crazy, but sometimes thoughts just fail to come as clearly as they used to. Occasionally, I would forget things that I would normally not forget. Also, I might be talking to someone, then get to a point where I just couldn't find the word that I wanted to say next. To the other person, this looked like I had lost my train of thought for a minute. In essence, I guess that I had.

Since the onset of my CFIDS, my thoughts do not flow like they used to. As a matter of fact, the writing of this book took me more than twice the time that it normally would have. I do not feel that I have developed any type of mental disorder and I do not lose touch with reality. Is that what some of the skeptics want to hear? Whether anyone believes it or not, this is a real symptom of CFIDS and I did not have it until I became ill with it.

I had always had some seasonal allergies. You know the typical runny nose and sneezing that normally only hits you during the spring. Well, that has become an animal within itself. Seasonal allergies appear to be in season all year long now. They had magnified twice from what they used to be. I realize that there are medicines for this, but I simply refuse to take any additional pills. I am already a walking pharmacy at this point.

Speaking of pills, I now have high blood pressure and borderline cholesterol problems. I really never had any such troubles until I got sick. If you noticed that I mentioned how I worked out all of the time and ate right, it seemed that I should not have those afflictions. I realize that both of these could be hereditary, so maybe it is not fair to blame it on the CFIDS. The only reason that I mention them is the fact that they both showed up when I got sick. Is there a connection?

Let's discuss aches and pains a bit. I have been afflicted with arthritic pains for years. Ever since I came home from service in 1991, it has been horrible. That has now increased in severity. As a matter of fact, there are new types of pains that have hit me since I became ill. It appears that I now have pains in my muscles and tend to injure them more frequently than normal. If you remember, I told you that I had studied martial arts for years. Since I was in the sixth grade, I have studied American Karate, Tae Kwon Do, Kung Fu, and Jiu Jitsu,. Many of these, I researched and tried myself, while many were taught to me by master instructors. I even had the privileged of spending a Jeet Kune Do training session with one of Bruce Lee's best friends.

At the age of thirty two, I was able to do a full split and throw a side kick nearly eight feet in the air. Now, that has left me. For something that has taken me twenty years to attain, it sure left me in a hurry. My muscles will not stretch the way that they used to. Once again, I know because I have tried over and over again.

You should be seeing a pattern in my behavior or my response to this illness by now. Every time that I tell you that I cannot do something, I mean it. That did not come from simply giving up or thinking that I could not do it, but painful trial and error. You see, I am not the type to give up and fold my hands. If someone tells me that I cannot do something, I will always prove them wrong. As mentioned above, I have finally met my match. That is not to say that I am going to stop trying, it simply means that I have proven the severity of this illness by experimentation. I don't like the results that my tests have shown.

CHAPTER 5

▼

YOU LOOK FINE TO ME

Welcome to the chapter that I could not wait to write! I believe that any of you that suffer from an illness such as CFIDS or fibromyalgia will enjoy reading this. Simply put, this chapter was inspired by the utter frustration with chronic fatigue and the reactions people give you when you tell them what you have. You may find that my writing in this chapter reveals a hint of aggravation. You guessed right! I tend to vent on paper at times, so bare with me.

I have heard people refer to Chronic Fatigue and Immune Dysfunction Syndrome as an invisible illness. Why is this so? Let's capitalize on that idea during this chapter. In some cases, it may not be, but all in all it is practically invisible to everyone else. When I say invisible, I mean the fact that the medical community does not have a standardized test to screen you for CFIDS nor is there a magic bullet to make it go away. So, it should not exist, right? It sounds crazy, but I still believe that it is looked upon this way.

There are organizations that are working very hard on the problem and from what I hear, they are doing a fine job. I am speaking more so along the lines of standard blood tests that you would encounter at your doctor's office. I am sure that if you dug deeper into the research world of CFIDS, you may find someone who could provide you with very impressive studies that show that chronic fatigue patients do in fact have metabolic changes going on within their bodies. How many of us who become ill, are going to be that fortunate? The average person, who becomes ill, simply goes to their family doctor to find out what is wrong. If your insurance works like mine, which is an HMO, you aren't going to convince them to pay for elaborate testing!

Just being realistic, most of us must seek medical help within our home towns. If you don't have a doctor who is knowledgeable about CFIDS or sympathetic to those afflicted with it, you may be in trouble. I was one of the fortunate ones. My doctor has been very helpful, and told me that medical science is still seeking the answers to this disorder. My specialist was also extremely sensitive to my condition. For that, I thank the good Lord above! So what does this have to do with CFIDS being an invisible illness?

As mentioned above, there generally are no standard tests available. Sure, there are theories such as the Epstein-Barr virus, but I think that they have even debunked that one. That was the only positive test that I had, by the way. Science seems to revolve around only what can be proven. If it cannot be proven, then the idea is questioned. Medical practices are no different. If a test shows normal, then there appears to be no reason to treat or diagnose something that is not there. This is where having CFIDS is very frustrating. In all honesty, I cannot blame doctors. If you test someone for practically every known illness via blood work, and nothing shows, what do you do? I believe it is also frustrating for doctors.

Until a test is developed for CFIDS, the doctor has to rely upon the word of the patient. Certainly, your symptoms may manifest themselves. For example, you may get recurrent infections that do show up on a test. I am talking more about a general test for the disease as a whole. Hopefully there will be one day. Otherwise, your doctor has to make a choice whether to believe your symptoms or not. This is where it is helpful to have a doctor that is familiar with the disease. You may have trouble convincing the skeptical doctors what is wrong with you, since you may look just fine.

I have had countless people tell me how well that I looked. Don't get me wrong, I am very fortunate to have so many family and friends that care. It is not so much that I want them to tell me how bad that I look, as it is that I want them to just believe me. None of my personal acquaintances have told me that they didn't believe I was sick Knowing how hard-core that I was before hand, the sudden changes in my lifestyle spoke for itself. You may have it harder.

The only time that I really *looked* sick was during the initial onset of the illness. Some of my fellow officers commented on how I looked very pale and sickly. At that point, they were right. But soon after the onset, my color came back and I began to look like myself. My weight, which had dropped rapidly by thirteen pounds, had climbed back to my normal range plus three pounds. I was able to do just enough physical activity to maintain my muscle mass, so I didn't look awful. It wasn't easy, but that is what I wanted to do.

Otherwise, you may have people tell you that you look fine and find it hard to believe that you have such a debilitating illness. One of these people may even be your doctor. This is the where the frustration comes in. For those of you who have experienced this, I am sure that I'm preaching to the choir! Unless you are completely bedridden, as many are, you may not show any outward signs of being ill. Fatigue doesn't necessarily make you turn colors, stomach aches don't change your appearance much, and brain fog can be a very quiet disorder if you don't talk to anyone much.

Maybe this is why the legitimacy of the illness is questioned so much. First of all, no one can seem to find a test that shows them that you have it. Next, the patient often times looks like a healthy person. I am a fairly muscular man. That comes from hard training and long workouts in the past. People may look at me and think how physically fit I must be. They may think that I am the healthiest person in the world. If they could only swap skin with me for a while! They have no idea that behind this healthy looking body, there is a man who has given up his career and countless activities that he loves to a hellish illness.

I don't know about other folks with this illness, but I have some good days mixed in with my bad days. They are rare, but they do come at unpredictable moments. I can't really get up in the morning and tell you if I am going to have a good day or not, as it just happens. Often times, it depends on what I did the day before. I meant to mention that earlier, but post exertional malaise may last for days after a strenuous activity. Anyway, there may even be just hours during the day that I feel better than others. I tend to try to make up for lost time during these periods and end up paying for it later.

It seems that during the good days, people have more of a chance to come in contact with you. On a good day, I will make my trip to the grocery store. In my home town, it is hard to go out without seeing someone you know. I will speak to these people and all that they see is that I was out shopping. You should see the look on their faces when I tell them how bad this illness is. I can almost hear their thoughts as they think how I must be exaggerating. If I was so sick, then why was I out buying my own groceries? I mean, sick people don't need food do they? Since I am sick, the world has to stop around me. The bills stop coming, the yard doesn't need to be mowed, and I have no need to get out of the house. In all practicality, I should be lying flat on my back with tubes poking out of every orifice.

It might sound hilarious, but don't be surprised if many people think that way. When you tell someone that you have a disabling condition, they immediately assume that you should be in a wheelchair or confined to a hospital bed. Truthfully, there are many with CFIDS that do indeed fit those categories. I am thankful for what I am able to do. I am sure that people with some terminal illnesses face some of the same problems. I have seen cancer and HIV patients doing more than some well people do. The problem with CFIDS is that it doesn't, and hopefully never will, fall under the category of a terminal illness.

The things that people don't see are the very things that disable people with CFIDS. When you are not at the grocery store trying to go on with your life, people don't see the suffering that you are experiencing. They don't know about the sleepless nights. They don't feel the joint pains in the mornings. They don't understand what it is like to search for a word, but realize that you have forgotten what something simple is called. They don't know what it is like when you come home from the grocery store and crash on the recliner because carrying the basket at the store was too much for you. They don't know how easy it is for your good days to disappear and become only a clouded memory. They just don't know.

To help you explain how rough this disease can be upon a person, let me explain something further. When I say good days, I am talking about good days in the present tense. I am not talking about feeling like I did before I got sick. Even though you may be having what you call a good day, it really isn't a normal day. They are still two different things. Before I got sick, a normal day was filled with anything that I wanted to do. Now, a good day is simply a reduction in symptoms just enough to allow you to increase your activity only for a brief period. In other words, once you begin to adjust to the illness, if there is such a thing, you develop a new definition of feeling good. My state of feeling good today would have been like feeling bad when I was well. If it sounds confusing, maybe you're right, but stay with me.

To help demonstrate this, I will use another personal example. One day I thought that I was feeling better. My throat was sore as usual and my neck glands were swollen, but I didn't feel any worse than I normally do. My fever began to climb, so I thought I needed to go to the doctor to check it out. I thought it was just one of those things. I tested positive for a strep sore throat and didn't even know it! I don't know how many of you have ever had a strep throat before, but I can tell you that they will put you on your back. I was simply feeling like I have felt continuously since I was diagnosed with CFIDS. The strep throat was simply hidden within my normal symptoms. The funny part was the fact that I thought that I was having one of my good days! Hopefully, you can understand what I was trying to tell you!

Another problem that fits into this chapter is the subject of disability. While many people are fortunate enough that their illness doesn't limit their work days, many are not as lucky. I am one of the unfortunate ones that have become unable to work on a full time basis since becoming ill. It was not my choice to get sick and I feel very bad about not being able to do what I loved. As a matter of fact, it feels like a part of me has died. Having severe symptoms and working do not always go together.

Certainly, it depends upon the type of work that you do and the severity of your CFIDS. Everything that I mentioned in this chapter can create a problem if you become unable to work. Let's say that you progress to the point that you are unable to do what you used to do. As a matter of fact, it is quite difficult to remain consistently well enough to do much of anything if you are severe. Now, you may have a doctor that doesn't subscribe to the idea of CFIDS, plus your employer thinks that you are lazy. Can you see the frustration building? Then you decided to apply for disability. That is a whole other battle within itself. You don't look sick. How could you be disabled?

I watched a very well made video about CFIDS called, *I Remember Me*. If you have not seen this, I would whole heartedly recommend it. On that video, several members of the general population were simply asked what they knew about Chronic Fatigue Syndrome. I was shocked at some of the answers people gave. I know that this doesn't necessarily represent the whole population, but it still got to me. Most of the people didn't have a clue, but others gave some wild answers. One person stated that they thought that CFIDS was something that only overweight women contracted! Another said that it was a mental disorder and that it doesn't really exist. Another stated that it was something that HIV patients got. I know that the above answers sound almost ridiculous, but they were real.

Some of my own friends even admitted that they thought it was a joke until they saw what it did to me. I think a lot of the problem is simply establishing more credibility to the illness. While on that thought, I can say that there is one organization that is very active in promoting public, as well as medical education regarding CFIDS. The CFIDS Association of America has invested millions of dollars in research, plus public awareness about this serious disorder. A breakthrough in helping others recognized the seriousness of this illness occurred when the CFIDS Association of American released the first public service announcement featuring former U.S. Surgeon General Dr. David Satcher. Visit their website at www.cfids.org to learn more about this outstanding organization, of which I am a member.

I told you earlier that even I had been a skeptic long ago. Still possessing the Army drill sergeant attitude, my answer to something called chronic fatigue was to get on the ground and push the laziness out of you. I knew of many ways to *motivate* an individual to want to end his or her fatigue! After being stricken by this inner enemy, my attitude has changed completely. I had met a foe that did not respond to my old way of thinking. My hardcore, sweat-it-out, get your head out of your—, attitude did not work this time. This was real and it had gotten hold of me.

So, how do you deal with looking great, but feeling horrid? How do you explain to family, friends, and coworkers about your illness? What if your doctor is not sympathetic to your illness? I wish that I had a magic answer to handle all of these questions for you, but I don't. I will tell you that taking one thing at a time helps. Trying to deal with your illness, plus convince everyone else that you are not faking symptoms can be difficult. Don't give up!

I am not telling you to give up your family doctor or giving you medical advice, but if you feel like you have developed CFIDS, then you need to see someone who has experience with it. Don't try to diagnose yourself! If you are becoming ill, go to whoever you are supposed to. If they tell you that all is well, but you aren't, then seek another opinion. No one can take responsibility for your health but you. It is my belief that there are probably many people suffering from CFIDS that are not diagnosed.

If your family or friends do not understand your illness, then educate them. There are plenty of resources out there on the subject that can help you with your explanation. Of course, this is only if you are definitely diagnosed with CFIDS. With the right doctor and plenty of your own research, you can help your peers understand why you feel the way that you do.

On the other side of the coin, who cares what other people think? Don't get so caught up in trying to prove to other people that you are suffering. Believe me, those that make fun of you or accuse you of lying need to watch out. From experience, CFIDS is no respecter of persons. Keep your chin up and your prayers flowing. You will make it!

In conclusion of this chapter, let me summarize what we have discussed. We looked at how there really aren't any tests that I am aware of that can diagnose you with CFIDS yet. Most tests simply rule out other illnesses that can mimic the same symptoms, which is important. We discussed the fact that even though you may be suffering from a very disabling condition, you may look perfectly normal. People may refuse to believe that you are sick, or simply think that you are faking symptoms, being lazy, or have a mental disorder.

I think that the frustration involved here is tough on the person suffering.

This subject deserves more exploring, but I will try to limit it to a few of my own opinions. During the course of my illness, I tried to read as much as I could about this illness. It seems only natural to want to learn about one's own affliction. The subject of questioning the legitimacy of CFIDS still astounds me. The opinion that CFIDS is simply anxiety or some other psychological disorder manifesting itself as an illness is simply hogwash in my opinion. The common denominator of folks making the suggestion seems to be that none have ever suffered with it. If they suddenly came down with a very real illness such as CFIDS, but no one could tell them what was wrong, do you think that they would settle for such an opinion?

Certainly I know that stress and anxiety can and does create real problems. I am not even a doctor but know that stress can make you physically sick. Many of us have experienced that at some point and time of our lives. How many times have you worried about an upcoming event, only to develop a stomach ache or headache? Being a former law enforcement officer, I know what stress is. I believe that some stress and worry is good. Without it, we wouldn't care what happened to us. Still, I think that one must draw the line somewhere.

While we all experience some stress in everyday life, we are not all disabled by it. Just as everyone with CFIDS are not all victims of excessive stress. From what I have read, there could be several hundred thousand people affected by CFIDS in the US alone. Are they all simply overstressed and manufacturing the symptoms themselves? A statement such as that is certainly silly. I can't speak for everyone, but I feel very comfortable in saying that I personally am not sick simply because it is in my head.

I tend to think this way due to my own will to get well. On a daily basis, I push myself to beat this illness. Everyday, I have the drive to get rid of it and continue on with my life. It has indeed put several speed bumps in my path since I became ill. With my positive attitude and my actions, I am persuaded that if it was purely mental, I would have beaten it by now. You may disagree and that is okay. That is what makes America a fine place to live! We can all share our opinions. I should hope that by now, you know what my opinions are on this particular subject.

We have mentioned that is an invisible illness can and does disable many people. Trying to find a doctor who is sympathetic, as well as gaining support from family offers other challenges. Living with CFIDS is quite taxing and very real. I don't think that it should be taken lightly by the medical community. From my own experience, I can honestly say that this so called invisible illness is a real whopper.

CHAPTER 6

▼

MY BATTLE STRATEGY

As I mentioned earlier, this chapter will deal with how I am fighting back against CFIDS. Once again I must remind you that this is only what I personally have done. I am not and cannot legally recommend you to follow any of my actions discussed herein. I do recommend that you consult your doctor before beginning any type of personal program that involves physical activity and/or nutritional supplementation. Without any further introduction, let's discuss my plan of attack.

I have a fairly extensive background in the realm of alternative healing. For the last ten years, I have studied every book that interested me on the subject of herbal medicines and holistic healing. I learned a great deal when I took the Doctor of Naturology course through the American Institute of Holistic Theology. My great grandfather was a healer and practiced many Cherokee methods of healing, so it just seemed to run in the family! Anyway, once I became ill, it dawned on me that I was going to try to beat this awful disease with the knowledge that I already had.

In addition to herbal preparations, I was a fitness nut. For the last seventeen years, I had been on some type of exercise program. Whether it was running, bodybuilding, or martial arts, I was always sweating it out. That is one of the hardest parts of being stricken with CFIDS; I am unable to do those things like I used to. Combining what I knew about both of these subjects, I set out to find the right healing program for myself. I dumped all of my reference books out on the floor and went to work.

From what I have read and experienced, a moderate exercise program can only be beneficial for my CFIDS. I will admit that there are some days that you absolutely cannot force yourself to exercise. If you really knew me, that statement would floor you. I have always been the type that would rather workout than do anything else. Unfortunately, my lifestyle has changed a great deal. In any rate, I still decided to keep a moderate workout plan. Actually, I should call it physical therapy instead of working out!

I designed myself a new workout program and kept a log of what I was able to do and when. The exercise program was very simple. In days past, I would have fallen asleep while doing this, but now it was like running a marathon! My program's equipment simply consisted of a level grassy field behind my house and a bamboo mat for the ground. I didn't even have to pay $60 a month to a gym! Other than that, all I needed was enough energy to use it and the motivation. The later was always there, but you can guess about the energy part.

Remember that CFIDS patients tend to have good and bad days. They both can be somewhat unpredictable. On my good days I would dedicate a few minutes to my exercise program. On my bad days, I just tried to survive. Anyway, I doubt that my old way of thinking was worth much now. I told you earlier that my idea of getting well was to put the running shoes on and sweat it out. That just didn't work anymore, so I had to adapt. From my own experimentation, trying to exercise on bad days despite how you feel is a mistake. It seems that CFIDS does not respond to motivation alone. Contrary to what some people may think about us *lazy* people with Chronic Fatigue, trying to push yourself only makes it worse. Had CFIDS simply been laziness, I believe that I would have figured it out by now.

My workout began as simply walking around in a circle for about four minutes. Once I was over the initial onset of my illness, my weakness was at its peak and four minutes was my maximum. On all my good days, I tried to do this in the morning hours. I started my program in the summer months, so the heat was a factor to consider. Morning air tends to be much more pleasant on the lungs. After a few weeks, my endurance increased to about six minutes. In reality, that is pretty poor, but I felt good about it. You have to remember that I was a runner beforehand. Walking for just five minutes and feeling exhausted was ridiculous to me, but I kept doing it.

After about two months, I could walk for eight minutes straight at a fairly quick pace. At this point, I was ready to add some other aspects to my program. I placed my bamboo mat on the ground and used it as an exercise mat. I slowly began adding a few sit-ups and push-ups to my routine. When I say a few, I mean only a few. I was lucky if I could do ten push-ups on a day that I felt good. My arms would shake, but I kept pushing. Sit-ups were easier to me, so I tried to do more of those. Anyway, the fear of getting a pot belly kept me motivated!

Several weeks went by and my muscular strength improved ever so slightly. I was astonished at how slow my body was responding to exercise. Before getting sick, I could have been ready for a triathlon by now. My body just didn't want to improve no matter what I did. What few improvements that it did make, were very slow to come. I tried not to do too much. It is also notable to mention that often times, I either did my walking or my strength exercises, but not both in the same session. I found out that strength training, such as push-ups, drained me faster than walking did.

As time went on, I was finally able to use my pull-up bar again. I started out by doing one set of three pull-ups. That was a tremendous chore, but I worked on it weekly. I tried not to do that type of exercise but twice a week. For me, pull-ups were the most difficult. Some days, I couldn't do one, but on others, a set of three was okay. I mentioned above, it seemed like my muscles would not recover or repair as they once did. Normally, I could begin to show strength gains within two weeks or so, but now it was a whole different ball-game.

After several weeks, I was getting very tired of being so weak and I missed running. I couldn't stand it anymore. So one day, I decided to go jogging. I have property in the country, so a nice deserted dirt road was perfect for me. If I fell out, I wouldn't have to worry about being run over by a car! It was a fairly warm morning and obviously, one of my good days. I put my headphones on and took off down the road. I was out of breath and exhausted about 100 yards after that! My chest hurt and I couldn't seem to breathe very well. Angry at my illness and myself, I did it again. The same thing happened. I finally had to do what I had never done before, and that was fall out of a run. In all of the miles that I had pounded out in the Army, I had never stopped during a run. It looks like my record is over now.

I eventually started trying to jog on all of my good days. I completely put away the strength exercises for a while in order to leave room for the endurance training. Here again, in the past, my two or five mile run always ended with pull-ups, sit-ups, and push-ups. That was definitely a thing of the past. I was quickly learning the principle of *banking* energy. This may be something that you have already discovered, but it is true. I found out that with CFIDS, you have to ration your energy levels.

You may have been used to doing several things in a row, such as going to the grocery store after your mowed the lawn. That too is now a problem. I figured out that I had to plan my activities in such a way that I was not trying to do too many things at one time. I applied this principle to not only my exercise routine, but to every aspect of my life. If you have caught on by now, you should be seeing that having CFIDS really causes some changes in your life!

We are now up to my current situation. I now rotate my physical training routine so that I never do the same things several days in a row. I may try to jog for five to eight minutes one day, and then do a few sit-ups and push-ups the next. On bad days, there is no physical training. If I have several bad days in a row, then I don't workout for several days in a row. Also, it is good to remind you that often times with CFIDS, you tend to crash after exerting yourself. I am still unable to beat this. A bad day almost always follows a good day for me. I still tend to try to do too much on my good days, causing post-exertional malaise that may put me in the bed the next day.

The above basically describes what I have done physically to beat my illness. I continue working on it when I can and hope that my outer and inner strength will bring me back to my old self. I also have placed myself on a natural supplementation program, which I will discuss shortly. But first, I still have some points to make that are brought to mind.

It is now quite obvious that exercising brings about an increase in my symptoms. My neck and armpit glands become more painful, my headaches return, and occasional nausea plagues me from time to time. Granted, these symptoms can even appear when I don't exert myself. CFIDS is definitely very complex and strange. I am guilty of pushing myself even when I should probably be in bed. That is just the way that I have always been. I am sure that someone will want to scold me for that, but this is how I choose to be. I doubt that anyone could deny the fact that I do have the motivation to beat this. This brings us back to a subject that I mentioned earlier in this text.

It still appears that many doctors and members of the general public are convinced that CFIDS is simply the manifestation of stress and/or lack of motivation to get well. Time after time, I have heard people tell me that I need to get it in my head that I am going to get well and to keep pushing through it. From the deepest part of my heart, if I try any harder than I already am, I will be in the hospital with a heart attack. Motivation and the will to survive are not strangers to me. Why do so many people insist that this illness is in our heads?

I told a friend of mine the other day that if I was sick simply because I was stressed out, I would be better by now. With everything that I have done, including stepping away from my role as an officer of the law, I feel that it would have subsided. Unfortunately, it still remains. I do agree with the theory that the adrenal glands may have something to do with Chronic Fatigue. I don't agree that it is the sole cause.

I have read several books about CFIDS since becoming sick. I have gotten angry when reading some of them, with the above in mind. I won't give you the name of it, but one in particular really chapped my posterior. It was written by a doctor, who had not suffered from CFIDS by the way. He constantly referred to how to relieve your stress. He recommended several natural alternatives, as well as medicines that he used on patients. Each one was seemingly designed to relieve depression or anxiety. He kept saying that once you got over your stress, your CFIDS would begin to get better. Hearing people tell me that I am sick simply because of stress is stressing me out!

I am sure that once more research is done on CFIDS, there will be some new theories. Until then, I will keep doing what feels right to me. Just remember that my way may not be your way. Now back to the next aspect of my recovery program. I warned you earlier that I would place my thoughts on paper as they arose!

Aside from my physical rehabilitation, I added a series of natural supplements to my diet. Actually, I should say that I added additional supplements to my diet, as I have always used some supplementation for the last several years. I do believe in the power of herbal medicines, as my ancestors relied on them completely. While some of my supplements were indeed used by the Cherokee, most are new. You may disagree with the amount and the dosage of what I used, but it is what I felt would work.

You should remember that even though you can purchase herbs and other preparations over the counter, they can have side effects. If you are taking any form of medication, be careful what you use.

You should always consult your doctor first. The reason is simple; herbs are simply a natural form of medicine. They have been used for thousands of years. They can react with certain medications that you are on, so pay close attention to what you are doing.

Simply for informational purposes, I will give you a run down of what I have used. This isn't a how-to book on herbs, and I am not making any medical claims. Look at it as simply my diary of what I did. You may already use natural supplements or some other form of holistic healing. There are many different options available. From acupuncture to massage therapy, the sky is the limit. I don't know if everything works or not, but if you are like me, you'll want to do whatever it takes to get well.

I also want to make it perfectly clear that I do not personally sell the supplements mentioned in this book. If I ever decide to, they will have to be something special that has really helped me a great deal. Otherwise, the information is simply to help illustrate what I do for myself. Often times you will read a book that is to supposed to educate you about a particular subject. Very conveniently, there is often an order form included where you can purchase everything that was mentioned in the book. You may also be directed to a particular place to purchase the products. From a marketing standpoint, that is pretty good advertising. However, I don't think that is always appropriate. This often makes it appear that the author was more interested in selling you his products than providing you with information that you sought when buying the book. I don't know about you, but wouldn't you write good things about a product in your book if you were selling it on the side? Almost makes you leery of trusting the author's word. I just wanted to make it clear that I do not sell the items mentioned, and will not try to convince you to buy anything. On particular supplements that may interest you, I will be happy to share with you where you may be able to obtain them, but I have no financial interest whatsoever.

The first substance that I use on a daily basis is Spirulina. I have actually used this for over seven years, but have recently increased my intake during the course of my illness. Spirulina is a form of blue-green algae that is normally commercially grown for human consumption. Don't go out to your neighborhood pond and scrape the top! My buddies always accuse me of eating *pond scum*, but that's really not what it is. Spirulina is actually a very nutritious substance. It contains a great deal of chlorophyll as well as protein and vitamins. I'll have to warn you that it takes some getting used to. Often times, the first few days of eating Spirulina can be somewhat uncomfortable. Your body has to cleanse and adjust to eating such a wild food. After a while, you'll get used to it.

I normally purchase the capsules, but have switched to the powdered form in ½ pound bags. I found this easier when it came to sprinkling it on food or mixing it into a protein shake. My average intake of Spirulina is about nine to ten grams per day. Most often, I simply take a quarter teaspoon with each meal. I have found that this supplement alone has always given me a subtle boost in energy. It doesn't contain any caffeine or stimulants, but simply nutrients. It doesn't make me jittery, but gives a very natural energy increase. Some folks take it before meals and claim that it helps decrease the appetite. That is one aspect of my life that has never left me!

The next supplement on my list is Alfalfa. This too has been a part of my diet even before becoming ill. Alfalfa is high in chlorophyll and minerals. I normally use about six tablets per day. You can also get an extract form that requires much less and appears to be more digestible. I added this for a natural mineral supplement and for it's supposed ability to help detoxify the liver. It has also been said that this substance is a good chelation agent. The most notable side effect that I noticed with this supplement was an increase in urination. It appears to somewhat of a diuretic. If you choose to use anything such as this, be mindful of your water intake and any other diuretic medicines that you may be taking.

Another supplement that I use contains immunoglobulins. It is sold under several trade names, but most appear to be about the same. I looked into the reasoning behind this supplement and decided to give it a shot. It is purported to help the immune system. At this point in my life, that is surely what I needed. I added one or two capsules per day of this. Currently, I cannot honestly say if it is actually making a difference or not. Time will be the judge. As far as any side effects, I have experienced none.

I also added L-Lysine to my regimen. I did this specifically for the ulcers that I have been plagued with in my throat. Since coming down with CFIDS, the ulcers are very frequent and extremely painful. I had learned that many people obtained relief from herpes outbreaks when using this. I had also heard of other people that had throat ulcers using it with great success. I started out with three 500 mg tablets per day, and then tapered down to one a day. It appears that I am having fewer occurrences of the throat ulcers with this supplement. Could it be in my head? Probably about as much as this whole illness is.

The next supplement on my list is Dandelion root. Yes, this is the same thing that grows in your yard and makes you angry. I added this supplement at the rate of about two capsules per day for the liver cleansing benefits. It is said that this herb is used to detoxify the liver. Since I have used several medicines and simply been as ill as I am, this couldn't hurt. I don't take this all of the time. I normally cycle it on and off. It is important to remember that if you are taking herbs, to come off of them every now and then. So far, all of my liver profiles have been within normal ranges. I haven't experienced any ill effects with this herb.

Since I have had recurrent infections since becoming ill with CFIDS, there has been some antibiotic usage. As you may know, this destroys both infections and good bacteria. Therefore, I added two tablets per day of Acidophilus. I have found that my digestion improves when I use this product. I am lactose intolerant, so I always use a milk free version. This one works for me, but we're all different.

My next supplement is elderberry extract. There has been a great deal of hype concerning this herb and viruses. I have read some interesting articles concerning this and thought it may help. Since I have been told that the Epstein-Barr virus *could* be a suspect with CFIDS, I thought I would try this one. Also, that seemed to be the only test that showed a positive when I was tested prior to diagnosis. I take this one on cycles also. Normally, I use about one or two teaspoons per day with meals. The brand that I use is mixed with raspberry and it actually tastes quite pleasant. So far, no real miracles to report yet, but I am hopeful.

Finally, I incorporated three 500 mcg tablets of vitamin B-12, plus two B-complex tablets everyday. Besides making my urine turn bright yellow, it does appear to give me an energy boost, plus some appetite increase. I realize that most of this is being thrown out by my body, but I wanted to flood myself with it anyway.

This next item falls into a category by itself; therefore, I decided to keep it separate from my list of nutritional supplements. Being a martial artist for many years in the past, I had encountered something called Qigong. It is basically a method of harnessing the power of the chi or life force by utilizing both meditation and special breathing patterns. I had practiced this in the past and found some amazing results. It seemed that after practicing my deep breathing exercises for an extended period, I noticed an increase in energy and weight loss. It really made me feel good to practice this art form.

After spending some time looking into this unusual way of fitness and healing, I dug into what I thought made it do its thing. Don't get me wrong, I do believe in the power of chi and mind over matter, as I have applied that principle myself many times. On the other hand, what was this deep breathing really doing otherwise? It was saturating my system with oxygen, the most life giving substance next to water in my opinion. I decided to explore this principle even further in reference to my current situation.

I took this on by a two-way approach. First of all, I dug out my reference books on Qigong and began doing my old breathing routine. This was something that I tried to do everyday, but not always. You have to make it a pleasant experience and not feel like it is work. It feels good and it shouldn't be ignored by anyone, since we all tend to breathe improperly all of the time. The next part of this approach was to include supplemental oxygen. About fifteen years ago, I found a product in a sporting goods store that caught my attention...bottled oxygen. This gave me an idea.

First let me tell you more about this amazing item. This product that I had purchased was basically canned oxygen with a small mask attached to the spray nozzle. It was sold as a recovery supplement to use by athletes. You would simply place the mask over your nose and mouth and give yourself a little spray of oxygen. I know what you are thinking...this guy has gone nuts. He is buying bottled air. How about some swamp property in the Sahara Desert too? Just keep and open mind and stay with me. Also, keep in mind that normally oxygen has to be prescribed by your physician. Even if you decide to try a sports product, always check with your doctor, as this may not be appropriate for certain conditions.

Anyway, this non-prescription oxygen actually worked. When I would get overheated or tired after a long run, I would take a hit. My recovery time was decreased and I felt an increase in energy that I normally would not have had. This is where my idea came in. Since practicing deep breathing gave me energy and even a bit of weight loss, why wouldn't supplementing oxygen give me an added boost? I went looking for this same product, but evidently, this company wasn't around anymore or simply stopped making the product. However, I did find comparable products elsewhere.

A told you earlier in this chapter, this isn't an official endorsement or a commercial, so I will not mention the names. I do not sell these items, so don't ask. The products that I found were very similar and offered a non-prescription oxygen supplement in a pressurized canister. You simply spray and breathe. One of them actually had the mask that was similar to the same principle used by the older product that I had used before. One of the products was imported and apparently is somewhat popular overseas.

I began breathing this oxygen at various times during the day. I never took more than just a couple of breaths at a time, as you can get a slight headache if you get too much. Normally, I would use it after I did my daily or weekly, depending on how I felt, exercise sessions. Since becoming sick with CFIDS, I get short of breath quite easily and have found that hot days make it hard to breathe. I would suck down some of the O_2 and get an amazing response. As in the past, it appeared to give me a very noticeable boost in energy and recovery. I often times took some when simply doing nothing and found that it just gave me my breath back.

Just let me note here that I am not really having any breathing difficulty. I say that I get short winded and find that hot days make it uncomfortable, but I don't have any type of lung disease. You should keep this in mind if you are having breathing problems. This type of thing is not to take lightly. If you are experiencing real trouble getting your breath, get to the doctor.

So, my own personal experience with this new *air in a can* is actually quite good. It may not do a thing for you, but you know that we are all different. One interesting note here is that oxygen is becoming more popular than you think. A little searching on the internet will reveal to you that there are things called *oxygen bars* popping up here and there. An oxygen bar is similar to a nightclub, except you get to listen to your favorite music with a nose cannula draped around your head. Instead of alcohol, you may sip on a healthy herbal drink while you huff some O_2 that may be infused with various aromas.

I realize that I jumped off on a tangent here, but the idea was just so interesting to me, it had to be explored. You may still be thinking that I flipped my lid when I said that I was snorting air out of a can. Who knows? This could be a very popular item in the near future. With the ozone layer depleting, we may all need an extra whiff of oxygen one day. Hey, they laughed when people started selling bottled water! How many of you have never purchased water in a jug or bottle before? Just some food for thought!

As you can see, I chose my supplements according to what I wanted to work on. This is where natural healing and medicine often go separate ways. Sure, medicine is good and I have to use some medications everyday. I am quite thankful that we have the medical technology to alleviate illnesses that once were often fatal long ago. However, too often medicine seems to target symptoms and not necessarily the cause. I am sure that many will feel that this is an opinion, and you are right. I believe in both medicine and herbal preparations. In natural medicine, you target the immediate cause or cleanse the body as a whole to help stimulate your body to do its own healing.

This is another area that people get confused. Natural healing methods often do not work like medicine at all, but some do. That is why you have to be careful ingesting both and you need to make your doctor aware. Holistic healing tends to help your body start healing itself again. You cleanse toxins and give your body a break from the stress of everyday toxins. From refined sugar to fried foods, these alone put undue stress on your system. That is my goal with my own program, to help rebuild what is already there and hopefully feel well again.

On top of exercise and supplementation, I altered my diet somewhat. Granted, I have never really been much of a junk food addict. In the last fifteen years, I have always watched my diet somewhat. I was never so strict as to make myself miserable, but I didn't gorge myself on junk. People used to laugh at me and tell everyone that the only thing I ate was grass! A big exaggeration, but often times not exactly untrue. Since I became ill with CFIDS, I thought it was important to crack down even more.

I still binge every now and then, but I pay more attention than I used to. I began eating more raw vegetables, as well as steamed. I cut the fried foods out completely and make sure that I drink plenty of water. Soft drinks are a big no no! Besides sugar, some of the ingredients need to be labeled as poisonous. Well, you know that I am exaggerating, but just hear me I am not going to name it, but one particular soft drink can erode a nail if you leave it in there long enough. I don't care to put that in my stomach. As a matter of fact, we might be surprised to find out how many things that we consume regularly might have to potential to harm us over time. Anyway, simply cutting out soft drinks can help shed some of those unwanted pounds. This brings up a point that we should stop and discuss.

I have read several articles and reports that suggest that CFIDS patients tend to gain a considerable amount of weight during their illness, particularly at the onset. One source cited that gains of twenty to fifty pounds were not uncommon during the first year. I'm still straddling the fence on this one. I have heard others with CFIDS discuss that they lost weight at the onset. I was one of those folks as I dropped almost thirteen pounds without effort in less than a few weeks. Now, I have gained my weight back to my normal range, plus a few.

I am not sure about this theory, but there could be something to it, depending on the individual. If CFIDS affects the thyroid, it could cause weight gain or loss. One source stated that his patients gained weight due to thyroid dysfunction despite normal test results. You'll have to think about that one on your own. My thyroid profile has always been within normal ranges and I don't feel that this one applies to me, but it could to someone else. There could be other reasons for weight gain with CFIDS.

If you remember, I have stated several times that what I experience may be totally different from what you do. My specialist even told me that this illness affects people in very different ways. I guess that is where I had the problem when I read that one physician made it seem that everyone with CFIDS would gain tremendous weight at onset. You may have to take into account what the person's age and fitness level was prior to becoming ill. I guess that if a pro football player came down with CFIDS in contrast to someone who was already overweight, you may see a difference after onset. Who knows?

I would be a liar if I said that the above didn't spook me enough to further alter my diet. Although I was quite comfortable with my diet and fitness level prior to becoming ill, I didn't want to see myself gain fifty pounds! This was probably a needless worry, but it assisted in my motivation. My diet isn't unbearable and it's easy to follow. Basically, I just use common sense and space several small meals throughout the day rather than eating three larger meals. This was a principle that I followed when I was a fitness trainer and into bodybuilding years ago.

The idea behind spacing smaller meals out is two fold. One reason is that it helps to maintain a more balanced sugar level, thus assisting with energy levels. When you have CFIDS, this is extremely important, as my doctor reminded me. Second, it starts your metabolism several times per day rather than just three. In other words, when you eat a meal, your body goes to work digesting and all of that good stuff. Why not jump-start your body systems five or six times and increase the fat burning furnace? It sounds silly, but as a former bodybuilding nut, I can say that it is amazing. Keep in mind that you cannot eat six full meals a day and lose weight.

I eat at least three meals a day that contain more calories than my other two. My in between meals may be nothing more than a protein shake and some fruit. All that I am doing is spacing my daily caloric requirements into five meals. I do this by calculating my basal metabolic rate and dividing. Your dietician or doctor can probably help you with this.

There is one more important point that I wish to make before my conclusion of this chapter. From what I have seen on the internet, there are literarily dozens of so-called cures for CFIDS out there. Many are attached to companies that are only out to make the money. Be careful what you decide to look into. You should also note that many advertisements tend to walk the border on illegal claims when trying to sell you something. As sad as it is, some people would rather make the money than care about your health. I chose most of my supplements due to past experiences with them or simply researching each one by itself. All I ask is that you be careful with advertising scams when it comes to this topic.

I will have to be honest when I say that CFIDS patients are the best to prey on. We are all desperate to get well and we feel horrible. That tends to make us a bit more open minded to some of these claims to healing. At one point, if someone would have told me that eating dried mosquitoes off of a car bumper would have healed me, I think that I would have considered it. Just be careful!

In the realm of cures, I have read several articles concerning a new drug that is supposedly nearing the end of the approval process. I don't know a great deal about it, but what I can gather, it must be some type of immunostimulant drug. While this may be a promising development, I still tend to have apprehension about it. This is probably just a personal problem, but new drugs often tend to scare me a bit. I'm a little leery of medicines in general, although I have to use them everyday. My worries are usually alleviated with the test of time. After thousands of people use it safely, with good results, I tend to get more trusting.

In any other type of product, new and improved usually means something good. However, with medicines, new means that not many folks have had the opportunity to use them yet. I am aware that the approval process is quite lengthy and very expensive, but it still seems risky at first. Anyway, if CFIDS is such a complex illness with so many different symptoms, how can one drug even begin to scratch the surface? If a new drug is approved, on what particular affliction is it based? As we have discussed many times, no one has yet to give anyone a definite answer as to what actually causes CFIDS. If that is the case, what are you going to treat? It's just another one of my wild opinions, or is it?

There it is. This is my own personal program that I still follow to this day. It is nothing that extravagant or scientific. The main idea behind it is simply the will to win. I chose to follow these paths because there aren't any real specific treatments for CFIDS as of yet. Of course, many doctors who specialize in CFIDS have their own methods, but still nothing that is straight across the board. Until then, I will probably keep doing what I have revealed to you. So far, I still have not beaten my illness, but that is yet to be seen. Once again, don't do any of this unless your doctor is aware of it. Only you can be responsible for your own health.

▼

MY THOUGHTS

This chapter is a bit different from the rest of the book, which appears to be more formal. I wanted to include a section devoted entirely to my own thoughts and opinions surrounding CFIDS and what it has meant to me. Actually, the majority of this book has been pretty much my opinion anyway, less what facts that I did research myself and should be credited to the original sources. As a matter of fact, I'll probably just throw all kinds of things in here for your reading pleasure. It may seem that I am repeating myself somewhat, as I will review some particular subjects discussed earlier, but with more detail. There are several points that I only touched on during the first part of the book that needs more exploring. This chapter should serve that purpose well.

CFIDS as a whole certainly does deserve more exploring. I hope that professional researchers will continue to learn more about it and find a way to stop it. I realize that there are many other severe illnesses out there, such as cancer, aids, and leukemia. For those afflicted with these horrid illnesses, I pray that you too will find hope and healing. We cannot get so caught up with our own afflictions that we forget that there are so many people who suffer greater than us.

You may have gotten the opinion from reading this book that I feel that CFIDS is the worst illness that you can have and that I don't recognize the others. That was not my intentions. I am very aware of the sufferings of others, as some of those illnesses have stricken my own family. I have lost relatives to cancer and other disorders. I have seen the pain in their eyes and the suffering that seemed to almost welcome death.

I was speaking with my pastor one day when he came to visit me during my illness. I told him that while I was in the hospital on the cardiac unit that I saw so many people who were dying. I also reminded him of how many people that I actually saw die as a law enforcement officer. This brought a new light to my eyes. When I begin to feel down on myself for being ill, and begin missing all of the things that I used to be able to do, I simply think back on those images. Those images are something that you cannot relinquish from your mind.

It makes me thankful for what I am still able to do. It reminds me of all of the things that I have done in this life and to be appreciative of having been able to be there. So many people that I have seen leave this world, never had the ability, nor the chance to take part in the adventures that I have. If you are just feeling down on yourself, go visit the children's hospital or take a walk down the hallway at a hospice unit. I guarantee that you won't be the same when you leave.

So what is the moral of my story? Simply put, be thankful for what you do have. For all of us that suffer with CFIDS, we do have legitimate problems. From reading this book alone, you have seen just one person's story of how this illness affected him. If you don't have this illness, you should at least now have a better understanding of what it can do. Even though we do have problems, you can always find someone who is worse than you. I am also guilty of feeling like I am alone at times in my own private hell. All I have to do is think about other people that battle such greater challenges. My illness doesn't seem so bad after that.

Going back to chapter five for a moment, you should remember that this section discussed how CFIDS is somewhat of a hidden illness. That is to say that it doesn't always make a person physically look any different. Countless times I have been told that I look like the picture of health. I'm not beating my own drum, but prior to getting ill, I was in pretty good shape. I'm not a small guy, and certainly not a weakling. Years of hard training has helped to shape me up to what I imagined that I should look like. I gave up on the Hercules syndrome years ago when I quit bodybuilding. Having gigantic muscles doesn't impress me much anymore, as it slowed down my running. But all in all, I look pretty healthy.

As I mentioned earlier, that can actually be a problem for someone who has CFIDS. The problem is not with the patient themselves, but with their peers. Standing before a disability judge and telling them that you have a debilitating illness, while possibly looking better in shape than the judge is, can be confusing. I was guilty of that in the past myself. I often times looked at a person that told me they were disabled with an evil eye. I'm not talking about someone in a wheelchair or an elderly person, but someone like me...a person with an illness that I couldn't see on the surface. I would think to myself that this person must simply be scamming the government. I am ashamed of it, but that is how I used to think.

While growing up, my mother used to tell me to be careful what I said about someone else. She told me that it could always come back on me. Now, I can really understand that. Often times, people are suffering when you and I do not know it. Only God knows what each person is going through. This still causes us a problem. Most people do not want to hear you complain. If you do complain and tell someone every time something is wrong, you are a whiner. However, in the case of really being sick, if you don't complain and show the people that count that you are sick, you can be labeled as a liar. Keep in mind that I am specifically speaking about CFIDS when using these examples. Some illnesses are quite obvious and need no explaining, but Chronic Fatigue is quite different.

As I mentioned earlier in the book, who cares what other people think? That is true, but at times you have to prove yourself. This comes under the battle of disability for people with CFIDS. Many people who suffer with this may need to apply for their disability benefits. Since medical science still can't give us an objective test for CFIDS, it still appears wishy-washy in the eyes of review boards. Sure, it's recognized as a serious illness, but due to the lack of a blood test for it, they tend to doubt us somewhat. I guess that I can understand, since any old Joe could come up and say that he had CFIDS.

The hopeful side to this is the fact that there are places that are finding that certain elements can and do exist with CFIDS patients. We mentioned Epstein-Barr, recurrent infections, and others that *may* be the cause. I guess that they just have to learn to look at both the patient's history, as well as the body as a whole before determining whether the patient is honest or not. You have to remember that I have spent the last decade as an officer of the law. I can tell you for a fact that I have had my share of people lying to me! As in being a law enforcement officer, as well as dealing with a patient claiming a hidden illness, you have to know how to read the person. For me, I can just tell when someone is telling the truth. There are things that show up when someone is lying that make them undeniable.

This isn't a lesson on telling the truth, but it is very relevant. I have read how many people were indeed sick with CFIDS, but their physician and/or their loved ones thought it was either laziness or psychosomatic. Maybe I cannot speak for everyone, but my own battle with CFIDS is not in my head. This goes back to what originally led me to write this section. What if my family and other important people in my life do not understand or believe that I am really sick? I won't go back into this in detail again, so I would refer you back to chapter five.

My own experience with family and friends has been quite well, as I told you earlier in the book. My family physician, as well as my infectious disease specialist, have been outstanding and very compassionate toward my situation. I can only imagine what it is like for someone to be dealing with this illness, only to find that no one believes that they are actually sick. You may be one of those, and I ask you not to give up.

Even with the understanding of my family and friends, I wasn't surprised to find out how little most people knew about CFIDS. Although it is not really a new disease, information on it evidently has not been disseminated well over the years. For the most part, the people I know had heard of the term Chronic Fatigue, but knew little else. Even though I didn't do an official poll, I would dare to say that the majority of the population is probably in the dark about it. Hence, the other reason for this book.

The one thing that I did find out was that my friends and loved ones wanted to know more about it. Most of them told me that they cared to find out more since it has happened to someone they know. I think that this is a big factor when it comes to understanding of this illness. Often times anything can seem far fetched or unusual until it happens to someone you know. Then it hits home. I was proud that my friends cared enough to want to know more about what had happened to me. Many of them admitted that they had heard of CFIDS, but like me, thought it was a bunch of garbage. The elaborate change that it caused in my life made them take notice.

Think about this for a moment. I gave you my background earlier in the book. I explained how I was a former infantry soldier, drill sergeant, and a SWAT team member. All of a sudden, I have to give up everything in such a short time span. Knowing how law enforcement was my life, particularly the SWAT unit, made a big statement about what was going on with me. Why would someone with all of this going for them, suddenly throw it out with the trash? Why would someone who is lazy or had made up an illness in his head, give away all that he had worked for? I think you get my point. The details of my story may be different from others with CFIDS, but the situation is probably very close.

So what's the moral of this story? If you are suffering from CFIDS and you find it hard to convince others what you are going through, don't give up. Don't worry about what your peers think, because they are not the ones going through what you are dealing with. Keep in mind that people just don't understand this illness enough yet. Find a good doctor and educate your family. If your friends are truly your friends, they will not give up on you, so don't give up on them.

I mentioned in this book about the length of time that some have been ill with CFIDS. I can't tell you how long one could be sick with this. I have read accounts of people being sick for as little as two years to people being sick for life. I have also read how some people totally recover, and others relapse after a period of time. This is an individual experience that can vary from one person to the next. Since I am not a medical professional who is actively researching this, I cannot give you any specific details. All I can say is that it appears that the battle is long and tough; however, it can be won. Even though I still suffer from CFIDS as I write this book, I whole heartedly believe that I will recover. I'm too stubborn not to! It is my hope that you will keep the same motivation at the fore front of your mind at all times. I plan to write a revised edition of this book when I do recover. By that time, I hope to be able to share more information with you.

You may still be wondering if I had any idea as to why I contracted CFIDS. I touched lightly on this earlier, but I do have some more information to share. Although I have some theories, I really do not know for sure and cannot give you an exact answer. Most of my theories are just speculation or simply cumulative. However, one of my theories may get me in trouble for mentioning it, but I'm going to anyway.

If you remember from the chapter on my background, I told you that I had taken a series of vaccinations back in 1991. While processing into the Infantry Training Center, I received numerous shots and oral vaccinations. For the most part, we really didn't have a clue as to what we were taking. I do remember being told that one was the flu shot and another was a penicillin shot. In any rate, we took them all within a matter of minutes. I took them all and went on with my job. I didn't have any immediate reactions or local reactions if my memory serves me well. My short term memory is fading some with my CFIDS, but the long term seems to still be there. Go figure?

Within the next couple of weeks, I began to get ill. As a matter of fact, I was very ill. I felt as if I was getting a bad case of bronchitis and the flu. I had fever, chills, extreme chest congestions, and body aches. I coughed frequently and felt like I couldn't breathe when I went to bed. It got so bad one night that I went to the Army hospital emergency room. The doctor loaded me up with cough syrup and told me that I was having a reaction to the flu shot that I had taken weeks before. I accepted that and went back to my unit.

Almost thirty days had passed and I was still sick. It didn't feel like the flu to me. I was exhausted, feverish, and congested most of the time. Quite frankly, I felt like I had chronic fatigue syndrome. However, I kept pushing myself. After some time, the symptoms subsided. I came home in July of 1991 and went back to being a police officer at my old job. I was probably home for about two weeks when I noticed something in the mirror one day. My mouth was hurting and I went to the latrine in the police department to look. Upon opening my mouth, I noticed that the inside of my lips and mouth were starting to becoming ulcerated. There were little blisters popping up everywhere. This surely caught my attention. Before you begin thinking it, I didn't engage in any promiscuous relationships while in service. I was completely devoted to a young lady back home, believe it or not.

I noticed that I wasn't feeling so great, so I ended up getting some medicine for it. The doctor gave me a type of mouthwash to relieve the ulcers. That helped for the moment, but ever since, they returned at will. Most of the time, they appeared in the back of my throat. If you remember me mentioning this earlier, you should know that one of my current symptoms is ulcers in the throat.

From that point forward, it appeared that my immune system simply gave out. I was constantly getting sick. Every virus or flu that was in the air came to see me. I normally became so sick during these times that I couldn't work. It was becoming a problem for me and for my employer. It was something that I couldn't help. I went to doctor after doctor, asking them why I kept getting sick. Most would simply tell me that it was just the way my body was. Unfortunately for me, I didn't want to accept that. Besides, that didn't help me out much. As in my current situation, nothing really ever showed up on tests.

I battled this on and off until it became so severe, and then I was finally diagnosed with CFIDS. So what's my point here? Look at it as another opinion of mine, but my gut feeling tells me that it may have had something to do with the vaccinations. Keep in mind that many soldiers from the Desert Storm era have been diagnosed with the mysterious Gulf War Syndrome, which often does resemble CFIDS. From the studies that I have read, it appears that both deployed and non-deployed soldiers have exhibited symptoms. So what's the deal here? Your guess is as good as mine.

Another theory concerning my newfound lifestyle is that I don't believe that there are really any accidents in the Universe. From a Christian's standpoint, I know that all things are controlled by God above and his Son Jesus Christ. Many nights I have had discussions with the Lord about why he allowed this event to take place in my life. Notice that I didn't blame God, only questioned Him in prayer as to what His plan was for me.

Being a former soldier and law enforcement officer, I have been in situations that only could have been resolved by divine intervention. God has taken care of me in instances where it seemed very dim. I don't believe that He has turned His back on me now. If anything, maybe it was me that turned my back on Him. It appears to be human nature to whip out the old "why me Lord?" question when things are tough. That can often lead to self pity. Remember what I said above about visiting the hospitals? It is at this point that we have to get hold of ourselves. Like I said, I believe that God has all things in His control, even illnesses. It is easier said than done, but I try to remember that there must have been a purpose for allowing this to enter my life.

I'm not going to sit here and tell you that you have to enjoy being sick. I also believe that God wants us to be well and happy. He also gives us the knowledge and will power to do our part to get well. If we do our part, I believe that He will do His, if it is in his plan for you.

This brings up my next point. Since I have been ill, I have done something that I have seldom done in the last ten or more years. I have been still. I have taken time off from the busy world. Keep in mind that I hadn't planned to get sick and simply give up everything that was dear to me. Sometimes these things happen. I had to look for a positive side to it all. As I just stated, God may have decided that I needed this time for some reason out of my grasp. Therefore, I have seemingly stepped away temporarily from my normal lifestyle. You would be surprised how much you can change in such a short period of time!

I have used this time to not only seek answers for myself concerning getting well, but have used the time to reflect on my past. As I just told you, I hadn't taken time away from it all in a long time. It's common with most of us. We all lead very busy lifestyles. In the last hundred years, life has changed in many ways and some of it may not be good. Maybe we've started spending less time with our families and more time on the internet. Maybe we've stopped spending Sunday evenings with friends to get that extra bit of paperwork done for the job on Monday morning. The list in endless, but it has one thing in common. Our lifestyles are speeding up.

I don't want to confuse you by going back on what I stated earlier concerning stress, but this point is relevant. Even though I don't want to put the cause of CFIDS solely on stress, I do have the notion that it can play a part. Many of us are stressed and don't know it. Many of us may know it, but are ashamed to admit it because people might think I am crazy or depressed. It sounds silly, but think about it. We have become so accustomed to living a fast paced lifestyle that we simply accept stress and frequent illness as just part of living. We often look at it like paying bills. You're always going to have them, just learn to live with them. I don't think that we should be this way!

Even though I tend to get angry when doctors want to blame CFIDS solely on stress, it may be part of it. Some stress is probably good for you. It keeps you on your toes and careful. Too much stress can be harmful to your body. One theory that I have read concerning CFIDS was that it was caused by overworked adrenal glands. That probably isn't too far off, if it is true. In my opinion, anytime you overload something, it can give out. It you abuse your car and run it too hard while not taking care of it, the stress will take it toll. The human body is much more complex than an automobile, but the analogy is very similar. If we push ourselves to the limit, then take two more steps, I feel that we run the risk of wearing ourselves out.

From lack of sleep to pressure at the office, stress can take on many faces. You don't have to be confined to a mental institution or have some type of disease to be stressed. It is no respecter of persons. Anyone can become overstressed. You may be one that could simply change your lifestyle and find new health. Like I keep saying, I don't think stress is the only thing that can cause a person to become chronically ill, but it doesn't help much. Once again, if you know that you are over stressed, seek some help. Don't diagnose or try to treat yourself without help. This is serious business.

This brings us to my next point...a change in lifestyle. If you have been diagnosed with CFIDS, you will probably have to make some changes unless you are only afflicted mildly. As you should know by now, many are completely disabled from this illness. Many cannot get out of the bed. You can imagine the changes that they have undertaken. No matter the circumstances, a change in lifestyle may come for you. Just be prepared if you must do it.

I speak from experience on this one also. My life took an unexpected turn when I became ill with CFIDS. I didn't want to change, nor did I wish to give anything up. My mind wanted to do everything that I had always done, but my body simply wouldn't let me. Maybe we should call it the Mind-Body imbalance disease! I expect that others have felt the same way. One day you are leading a normal life, and the next you are struggling to get out of bed. That most certainly involves some very proactive changes.

This is another area that family, friends, and employers will simply have to understand. Although it may only be temporary, and I hope that it is for you, things may have to change. You may be able to still accomplish a percentage of what you used to do, but even that can be a challenge. I have every desire in the world to do on thousand things right now, but I can't seem to make them happen. This can create stress within itself, but you can overcome it.

With all of the above in mind, how has this really affected me? I realize that I included a chapter solely to the *new me*, but let's explore more. To try to sum it up with getting a bad case of diarrhea of the mouth, let's keep it short. In a word, I could say simply devastating. CFIDS has caused me to give up many things for now. Notice that I said the illness caused me to give things up, not a case of one simply giving them up. Simply put, I had to reduce my lifestyle to that of which I could handle without making me any sicker. It isn't fun, exciting, or very confidence building, but it's what I had to do.

If you paid much attention to my background, you can see that I am the type of person that likes to prove himself. I love to reach goals and find bigger, better things to accomplish. I referred to myself as a type A overachiever. That may or may not be true, but it sounded good! Anyway, I am the type of person that has to feel that he is earning his stay. If I don't workout, I feel like I'm getting fat and lazy. If I don't work, I feel like I don't deserve to rest. It may sound silly to you, but to me these things are real. They keep me motivated to do all that I can. Writing a book was a goal of mine that I have reached numerous times. Had I given up and told myself that I couldn't do it, I would have felt like a failure. Sometimes, my illness gives me the same type of feeling of defeat.

On the positive side, I am going to beat it. I am thankful for what I can do and give the good Lord above all of the credit. This has been a very devastating experience to me, but I look at it as only temporary. It is my hope that if you are stricken with CFIDS, you will keep the same attitude.

In reviewing the actual mechanics of dealing with CFIDS, I have found what makes me feel better and what makes me feel worse. I mentioned much of this in the chapter dealing with my battle strategy. To sum it all up for you, I'll tell you how it goes. I have found that strenuous exercise or any type of physical exertion does indeed activate my symptoms. In other words, should I be having what I describe as a good day, any exertion can change it to a bad day rather quickly. In this sense, maybe some aspects of my particular case of CFIDS are predictable. Other aspects simply come and go without warning.

I have found that moderate activity gives me a boost mentally and to a lesser degree, physically. As I told you in my battle strategy chapter, energy banking is quite important. While I still want to run several miles, and then end the workout with various strength building exercises, my body doesn't respond to that way of thinking anymore. Therefore, I have not only had to reduce my physical exercise program to nearly one quarter of what it was, I also had to reduce the actual number of activities that I do at one time. As I told you, the energy banking principle is now applied to every aspect of my life.

It is not easy going from one who is usually running a hundred miles per hour with his hair on fire, to one with the speed of a turtle.

As difficult as it has been, I am slowly adapting to a very new way of thinking. If I plan my exercise program in such a way that I only do one thing at a time, I have found that it agrees with my body much better. That is not to say that I still don't tend to crash my energy levels afterwards anyway, but it makes it more bearable.

In all honesty, do I actually feel that exercise, despite being sick, really helps? In my particular case of CFIDS, plus factoring in my former way of life, I would have to say definitely yes. I would be a liar if I told you that it makes me feel as good as it used to. More times than not, it makes me feel somewhat bad. You still have to remember what type of person I was or still am inside. I already had the discipline to push myself beyond what most would have done. That was just my way of thinking. I had already learned how to live with chronic joint pains in the past; therefore, I had the mindset to endure some more. I didn't say that it was easy. It's just what I want to do. If you suffer from CFIDS, you may not be able to do this. If you were out of shape prior to getting sick, it may be harder on you to start a program now.

In addition to a moderate exercise program, I have found that certain other things make me feel better and worse. Other than proper diet, rest is still important. Although with CFIDS, sleep doesn't always appear to relieve fatigue like it used to. I am speaking more along the lines of resting prior to becoming so exhausted. On days that I don't really feel like doing much of anything, I usually don't. I often feel that this is wasteful to simply do nothing, but at times it is the best thing for this illness. You have already found out that you cannot keep up the same lifestyle anymore, so here's another lesson to learn.

Since I figured out that activity can make my symptoms worse, I really use my feelings as a gauge to determine what I can and cannot do. If I wake up and feel that it is going to be a bad day, and often you can tell, I tend to be more sedentary. This is simply prevention. If I were to push too hard on a day like that, I can assuredly say that by the evening hours, I will be very sick. That is enough motivation to make me say no when I don't think that a certain activity is best.

Going back to the energy banking idea, even on good days you have to ask yourself whether something will be beneficial to you or not. If I feel more energetic, I will still be careful as to what I allow myself to do, simply of the fear of making my symptoms worse. It's not unusual worry, only learned behavior from trial and error. For example, if your cat bites you every time that you pet it, you'll probably think twice before petting it again. That's a crazy example, but is quite accurate when learning your own limits.

I dedicated a portion of the last chapter to my nutritional supplement regimen. In my opinion, I feel like it has helped me. I'm not claiming that the supplements can or cannot do any particular thing, but I feel benefits from them. The supplements that I have chosen have been very non-evasive and easy on the system. I feel that I may have gained one notch on the energy scale. It hasn't been anything dramatic, but enough to make me continue using them within reason.

You may be asking what my opinion is regarding CFIDS and the medical profession as a whole. In other words, do I think that many doctors are simply discounting the validity of the disease and ignoring it? From a patients view point, do I feel nothing is really being done about it? To answer these types of questions, you may want to hold on and read the last chapter which I wrote for the medical professionals themselves. Otherwise, I'll give you a hint as to what I think.

While I do agree that some doctors may be quick to jump the gun and say it is simply all in the patient's head, I don't believe that is the case in general. From what I have experienced and studied, there are more and more doctors becoming informed and involved in the battle against this illness. Now don't get the simple lack of information and total disbelief confused. Those are totally different aspects.

In other words, just because your family doctor doesn't have all of the answers, doesn't mean that he doesn't understand your condition. You may run into some here and there that are still headstrong as to what the real cause of CFIDS is, but generally you will be okay. I often like to compare police officers and doctors in certain ways. As an officer, I may work a case that is quite confusing. I know for a fact that a crime was committed, but I don't know who did it yet. It then takes a long time to get all of the facts. But to be thorough, you have to go through the steps. To some of my "customers", that may make it appear that I either don't know what I'm doing or that I don't care. They may not know what I do on my own when they are not around.

Try to look at the mystery of CFIDS and your doctor as being in the same boat. He or she may be totally convinced that you are sick, but unable to find the cause at the moment. Just like with investigating a crime, illnesses have to be investigated. Evidence must be gathered, tested, and proved before you can present your findings. In the mean time, we must simply stay cool and deal with it the best that we can. I don't think that trying to blame anyone else for you being sick is the answer. Sure, we all want answers and to get well, but we need to understand that having CFIDS is no easy task to deal with. Both you and your doctor are in it for the long haul, so be good to each other!

There is one other point that I wish to throw in here. I may have mentioned it briefly in the book, but I wish to go a bit deeper with this one also. The name Chronic Fatigue Syndrome simply doesn't do this illness any justice. It simply describes one symptom of the illness. Maybe this is one reason why many members of the public feel that it is garbage. Many people probably think that since everyone experiences some fatigue in their lives, then those of us who have Chronic Fatigue, have simply given in to it. There has been quite an uproar over the name and I agree. The name Chronic Fatigue and Immune Dysfunction Syndrome is becoming more widely accepted. At least that does give a bit more description of the illness somewhat.

I have heard that there is quite a bit of tinkering over the idea of coming up with yet another name. In doing so, they supposedly have to come up with a name that accurately describes the illness and does not solely focus on the fatigue alone. In my case, the fatigue is almost secondary to all of my other symptoms. Whereas fatigue is one of the symptoms which appears to be present most all of the time, many other symptoms wax and wane. How can you accurately describe an illness that is so complex? I wish them the best of luck!

As I begin to close this chapter I will offer those of you with CFIDS some advice that I feel quite safe in giving. First of all, if you are diagnosed with CFIDS, learn all that you can about it. If you are up to it, scour the internet for articles, and read some books. When you first come down with this illness, you may feel like you are battling alone. I can honestly tell you that you are not. There are many people with the same affliction with you, so don't feel lonely. Taking the time to educate yourself and your loved ones will help you to better understand what is going on.

You should talk to people. Don't keep your doctor or family in the dark! Let them know what is going on with you. Your doctor needs the information in order to help you. No one can read your mind. I'm not telling you to complain to everyone that you see, as nobody wants that. I am saying that you shouldn't bottle things up inside of you. That can make you feel worse. If you're worried, talk to someone you trust like your pastor or a close friend. If new symptoms appear or you get worse, let your doctor know. By learning all that you can about CFIDS, it will become less frightening to you. I can tell you that it can be scary if you don't understand what is happening.

If you are able to do so, try finding a local CFIDS support group. You will be surprised how many have sprung up across the country. This goes back to what I stated above. You can talk to other people who are experiencing many of the same things that you are. It's a great way to make new friends who will most certainly understand you! Visit my website for some information that can get you going on the right track.

If you are able, try to keep a log of your symptoms and your daily activities. This can have several uses. It can help you document your illness better if you need to apply for disability, plus it can be helpful to both you and your doctor. If you are able to go back and look at how you felt after doing a certain task, you can better plan your activities in the future. I have a log that I enter something in at least a couple of times a week, if I can remember to do it. It's nothing fancy, but just a list of how I felt and what I was able to do that day.

The next advice that I can give you is to find something that you enjoy doing that you are able to do. This may be an old hobby that you put away years ago, or it may be something totally new. I realize that when you are very sick, it is hard to do much of anything, but give it time. You may find that you always wanted to write a book or maybe start reading more books. Have you ever thought of learning to play the guitar? No matter what it is, just find something that gives you a goal and the will to do it. Once you find something, you may discover that it helps keep your mind off of simply thinking about being ill, which brings up another point.

I know that I have mentioned researching CFIDS and talking to people about how you feel. The one important thing to remember when doing all of this is to not let yourself dwell on the subject. The idea is to set your mind at ease, not stimulating additional worry. In other words, try not to think about being sick all of the time. I know that this can be hard, but try. The more you can keep your mind at ease, the better. This is where the hobby comes in. It has absolutely nothing to do with being sick. It is something totally different. Just remember that when seeking a new passion.

My final words of advice are to just know your limits and get well! Don't try to overdo it. If anyone could have found a way to rush this illness out quickly, I believe it would have been me. Follow your doctors instructions and keep the faith. Do only what you are able to and keep that within reason. If you are mildly affected with CFIDS, consider yourself very lucky. Many people with this illness do in fact continue on with their normal lives, but with some difficulty. Others just aren't so fortunate. Remember to be thankful for what you can do. Although I am convinced that my illness is not in my head, I do believe that a positive attitude can only help.

CHAPTER 8

▼

FOR THE MEDICAL PROFESSIONAL

I have directed this short and final chapter toward the medical professional. I actually had planned to end the book before now, but thought this final word would be a good addition. For any and all physicians reading this text, I wish for you to lend me your ears for a moment.

If you have read this book in its entirety, then you should have a pretty good idea of what my particular case involves, less lab reports and the like. As stated throughout the book, I wanted this to be a reference text for not only yourselves, but to your patients. I realize that I am not a doctor, nor do I claim to have any particular expertise within this field. I do however have first hand knowledge concerning CFIDS. Unfortunately, I obtained it the hard way.

You may or may not be one with much experience in dealing with patients with this disorder. I cannot and do not blame anyone in the field that doesn't completely understand this illness. Just like you, those who are afflicted with CFIDS want to learn more. That could basically establish a good reason for this book alone. While this text does not include confusing statistics, elaborate lab results, or controlled studies, it does come directly from one afflicted with the disease in question. It is my hope that something I presented to you may help with someone that you may be treating. Also, maybe it would assist your patient in better understanding what they are going through. Being sick and feeling alone in the battle does no good.

If there was a general comment box that I could leave you suggestions in, my requests would be simple. Should you have one or more patients that you have determined to be suffering from CFIDS, I would ask you to be as understanding as much lies in you. I am not suggesting that doctors in general are not sympathetic, but have met some in the past there were. This disease is very complex in my opinion and there are numerous studies to be done in the future. Although there is always hope for the future, your patients need you now. Tomorrow can never come soon enough.

I would think that most any patient suffering from CFIDS would ask of you the same thing, and that is to simply listen with an open mind. Why do I say this? If you have caught it several times in this text, often times people are simply told that it is all in their heads. While that could be true in any variety of instances, I just don't think that it is the case one hundred percent of the time. Just as in a terminal illness, patients with CFIDS need understanding.

These patients will probably complain a lot to you. They may have to have numerous appointments with you, each time with a different complaint. They may present very complex problems to you that may not have an easy answer. What you can give them is an understanding ear and the best medical assistance that you can offer.

I admire all the men and women in the medical profession as I have a sister in the field and once pursued it myself. I can only imagine the difficulty that you experience when presented with a problem such as CFIDS, whereas no particular treatment has been established. From a patient's standpoint, we must also be understanding to your situation. In essence, I guess the understanding has to be two way.

My final suggestion to you would be that I ask you to learn as much as you can about this debilitating illness. As time goes on, you may begin to see more and more people exhibiting symptoms characteristic of CFIDS. It is my belief that knowledge is power. Certainly this situation is no exception. I have included a list of my references at the end of this book, which lists some very good places to start if you haven't already.

I would also hope that you find this book a good reference to advise your patients to read. When I wrote this book, I tried to think about what I would want to find in it myself. If I was recently diagnosed with an illness that neither I, nor my doctor knew very little about, I would want to learn more. Being sick is one problem, but being sick and in the dark is another. While this book isn't written by someone with a string of letters behind his name, it comes from the heart and hardcore experience. I tried to think of questions that someone with CFIDS would ask, and then answer them with my own experiences. You already know how important patient education is.

My own physicians were very honest with me concerning CFIDS. They told me up front that they did not know all of the answers to this complex illness. They informed me that there was plenty of research that needed to be done. I respected that much more than if they had tried to feed me a line of garbage simply because they were afraid to say that they didn't know. As in my days as a law enforcement officer, I always preferred people to be straight with me. Your patients will respect you much more for that.

Another point that I wish to mention is that you may have found my methods of dealing with CFIDS somewhat unorthodox. Not everything that I did would be accepted as practical by the standards of medicine. You may find that many of your CFIDS patients tend to follow similar paths. Why do we do this? There are several answers to that question. First of all, there is currently no particular treatment that you can offer for CFIDS. Next, your patients want to get well. This illness is severe enough that many of your patients may feel like they are slowly dying. I realize that there is little to suggest that this is or could be a terminal illness, but your patients know how they feel. The simple desire to get well and the will to win the battle may prompt them to ask you about alternative therapies.

I realize that as a physician, there are things that you may not be able to legally prescribe within the world of alternative medicine. However, if your patients make the decision on their own, I would only ask you to keep an open mind. Obviously, there has to be a ceiling there somewhere. Some alternative therapies do not mix well with needed medications that your patient may be using. Just remember that the patient just wants to get well. Just because no particular blood test exists as of yet, it doesn't mean that they are not suffering.

Finally, I want to remind you of something else. Often times I have compared doctors, law enforcement officers, and preachers as having much in common. They all serve the public in one way or another. Each one of these professions requires a great deal of understanding, as well as the ability to listen to others complain. That can be a trying experience. I have felt that strain many days as a law enforcement officer myself. Sometimes, the biggest problem could come from within when we feel that since everyone complains to us, they must not appreciate what we do. That is so far from the truth.

The fact of the matter is that you are appreciated for what you are able to do. From reading this text and maybe others about CFIDS, you may get the impression that blame is placed on the doctors for not knowing everything about it. I am sure that some people have or will become angry if you tell them that you do not know exactly how to make the well again. From my standpoint, I do understand and appreciate what the medical professionals have done or have attempted to do for me during my battle with this illness.

In conclusion of this section devoted to the treating physician, I hope that my book has been of some assistance to you and your patients. I stress again that I don't claim to have the answers or be some type of self proclaimed expert. If this book will help only one of your patients understand their affliction better and that they are not alone in their battles, then my goals have been accomplished.

CONCLUSIONS

▼

As we come to a close, let's take a look at what I've discussed with you. First of all, I tried to make it a point to all my readers that it is my opinion that Chronic Fatigue and Immune Dysfunction Syndrome is not all in our heads. It is a very real and debilitating illness that affects many adults and children around the world. In helping to make my point, I gave you a short autobiography of who I was prior to becoming ill. My main point was to show that I was not simply lazy and decided to give up on life all of a sudden. From what I have heard people say about this illness at times, it makes you think that some actually believe that is what many of us did.

I took you through my own personal experience with CFIDS, as I described exactly what it felt like when the initial onset struck. From every text that I have read on this illness that appears to be what was missing. Don't get me wrong, there are some excellent books out there and they did help me understand this disease better. The biggest problem with most was the fact that many authors did not tell you what it was like when they became ill. Others were doctors who had never suffered with it. I feel that someone who is or has dealt with this illness can better explain themselves.

We looked at how it changed my own life. If you think about it, the changes were pretty drastic. While some are lucky and are not struck as hard, many are brought to their knees. When dealing with CFIDS, we're not talking about a case of the flu or a stomach virus that will go away in a couple of days. You are dealing with a serious illness that can affect you for life. As I have stated in this text, I believe that this is one of the most devastating aspects of CFIDS. When one has to make major changes in their lifestyle, it definitely proves that it is nothing to laugh at.

I also tried to give you my perceptions of what I think CFIDS really is. If I knew, then I must be smarter than all of the researchers working on the problem today! In essence, all that I have done in this text is simply repeated what is already known, with a personal opinion twist. You can take that for what it is worth. It was written by a CFIDS patient for others with the same affliction, and anyone in the medical field that wants to read a self reported case study. I am sure that as time goes on, more information will come to light. Hopefully, a cure or specific treatment will emerge that is successful.

We looked at what I call my battle strategy against this illness. If you got the picture that I have taken the illness on head first, you are right! I simply did not want to sit back and just be sick. Whether my method works or not, at least that I was fighting the entire time. Sure, I suffer while I am fighting it. I just don't let my motivation go away. If I could offer you one piece of advice, that would be it. I'm not telling you that motivation will make your illness better, but simply stating that you are more likely to accomplish something if you keep your eyes on it. Who doesn't want to get better?

Finally, I shared my personal thoughts and observations surrounding CFIDS and how I perceived all that comes with it. In my opinion, chapter seven is probably the most important chapter to me. When writing this book, I left that chapter open so that I could put thoughts and points there that may not have fit elsewhere. It also gave me a chance to vent about a few subjects that deserved a bit more hot air!

You may have felt that I was over exaggerating many things concerning CFIDS and other topics mentioned in this book. You may have also got the feeling that I was being too harsh with some of my opinions. If you did, that is okay. If we all agreed on everything, this would be a dull world! On the other hand, I may not have been harsh enough on some subjects. All in all, I tried to show that even through my own frustrations, I am still sympathetic to both doctors and other people with CFIDS. As I warned you before, you could have detected a bit of anger in some of my chapters. That may have been the case. After all, having a chronic illness and dealing with everything that surrounds it, can be quite testing. Even writing a book can try your patients!

I hope that this book has enlightened you in some way. I know that it doesn't contain the magical cure, but hopefully the information was useful to you. If anything, I wanted the reader to simply understand what it is like having CFIDS. Besides the medical mystery that plagues our doctors, the general public still hasn't fully grasped what we suffer from. There it nothing more aggravating than to feel so bad and have someone not believe you. I would refer you back to the chapter titled *You Look Fine to Me* if you haven't caught that point yet.

If you are a medical professional, I hope that my book served as somewhat of a case study from a patient's perspective for you. The way I look at it, if patients share more with the doctors, then the doctors will eventually be able to share more with us.

I will probably attempt a revised version as time goes on. In that version, I hope to report my recovery from my illness. I don't know when that will be, but I am convinced that it will be. Thank you for being a loyal reader and if you are stricken with CFIDS, I pray that you will recover soon yourself. If you wish to share your comments about this book, I would be happy to hear from you. Please visit my website at **http://www chronicfatigue-book.com.**

About the Author

The author was born near Charlotte, North Carolina, and graduated from basic law enforcement training in December of 1989. He has spent the majority of his career as a law enforcement officer and with four years as a SWAT team member. He holds an associates degree in law enforcement technology, and has had two years of pre-med. study in Charlotte, NC. He is currently a member of the North Carolina Justice Academy Alumni Association.

He is an honorably discharged veteran of the United States Army Reserve, with training as an infantry soldier and drill sergeant. The author spends his spare time writing and creating Native American artwork. He and his mother, being of mixed Cherokee Indian blood, are enrolled members of the Echota Cherokee Tribe of Alabama, which is one of seven recognized tribes in that state.

Brian E. Voncannon has published five books prior to *Chronic Fatigue Syndrome: Living with the Unknown.* His most popular book was *Living Behind the Shield: A Modern Warrior's Path to Bravehood,* which entailed the experiences of being a law enforcement officer and the impact it has on officer's lives. This book gained him an appearance on a North Carolina television show, as well as an article in a national magazine.

Brian chose to write his current text after being diagnosed with Chronic Fatigue and Immune Dysfunction Syndrome. He felt that there needed to be a text geared toward the individual and medical professionals simply seeking to hear from a patient about what it is like to live with such a disorder. Brian hopes to revise the edition in the future.

Bibliography

Chronic Fatigue Syndrome Information Page: Center for Disease Control and Prevention. Retrieved July 2002 from the World Wide Web:
http://www.cdc.gov/ncidod/diseases/cfs/info.htm

The Possible Role of Vaccine Adjuvants in Persian Gulf War Veterans' Illnesses. Retrieved June 2002 from the World Wide Web:
http://www.gulflink.osd.mil/finalrpt.html

About CFIDS: The CFIDS Association of America. Retrieved on June 2002 from the World Wide Web:
http://www.cfids.org/about-cfids/default.asp

Chronic Fatigue Syndrome: UC Davis Health System. Retrieved June 2002 from the World Wide Web:
http://wellness.ucdavis.edu/medical_conditions_az/ chronicfatigue07.html

Vaccines May Be Linked to Gulf War Syndrome: ChiroWeb. Retrieved June 2002 from the World Wide Web:
http://www.chiroweb.com/archives/18/13/04.html

Balch, James F. M.D. and Phyllis A. C.N.C. *Prescription for Nutritional Healing*: Garden City Park, NY: Avery Publishing Group 1997 Second Edition

Colbert, Don M.D. *The Bible Cure for Chronic Fatigue and Fibromyalgia*: Lake Mary, Florida: Siloam Press 2000

Teitelbaum, Jacob, M.D.. ***From Fatigued to Fantastic:*** New York, NY: Avery 2001

I Remember Me Snyder, Kim A: Zeitgeist Video 2000

0-595-24182-4